NATURAL
MENOPAUSE

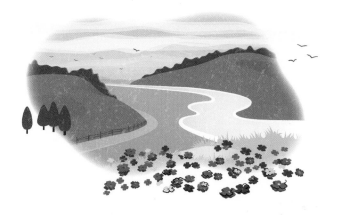

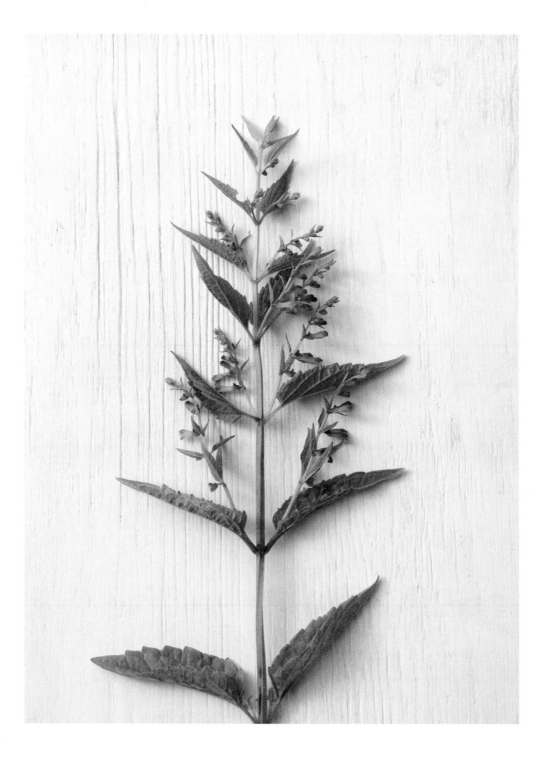

NATURAL
MENOPAUSE

HERBAL REMEDIES • AROMATHERAPY • CBT • NUTRITION • EXERCISE • HRT

Consulting Editors **Dr. Anne Henderson,** MA MRCOG
Dr. Rebecca Dunsmoor-Su, MD MSCE NCMP

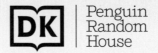

Project Editor	Claire Wedderburn-Maxwell
US Executive Editor	Lori Hand
Senior Art Editors	Emma Forge and Tom Forge
Senior Designer	Barbara Zuniga
Editorial Assistant	Kiron Gill
Senior Jacket Designer	Nicola Powling
Jacket Coordinator	Lucy Philpott
Production Editor	David Almond
Senior Producer	Luca Bazzoli
Creative Technical Support	Sonia Charbonnier
Managing Editor	Dawn Henderson
Managing Art Editor	Marianne Markham
Art Director	Maxine Pedliham
Publishing Director	Katie Cowan
Illustrators	Keith Hagan & Nicola Powling
Photographer	Ruth Jenkinson
Food Stylist	Tamara Vos
Prop Stylist	Robert Merrett

Disclaimer, see page 223

First American Edition 2021
Published in the United States by Dorling Kindersley Limited
1450 Broadway, Suite 801, New York, NY 10018

Copyright © 2021 Dorling Kindersley Limited
DK, a Division of Penguin Random House LLC
21 22 23 24 25 10 9 8 7 6 5 4 3 2 1
001–320990–Mar/2021

A catalog record for this book is available from the Library of Congress.
ISBN 978-0-7440-2690-0

Printed and bound in China
For the curious
www.dk.com

This book was made with Forest Stewardship
Council ™ certified paper – one small step in DK's
commitment to a sustainable future. For more
information go to www.dk.com/our-green-pledge

CONTENTS

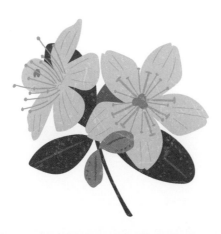

FOREWORD

Why a guide to "natural menopause"? As an OBGYN and menopause practitioner my constant refrain to my patients is, "this is a natural and normal process." I think reframing menopause as a normal and manageable transition can be beneficial for women.

It might seem unusual for a Western medicine practitioner to be involved in a book that primarily focuses on "nonmedical" interventions and herbal remedies. We have lost our focus in Western medicine, in my opinion, and instead of generating and supporting wellness, we often find ourselves playing catchup and treating illness. Don't get me wrong, I have a strong belief in science and the Western medical tradition. I am an epidemiologist by training and am most influenced by data and statistics. But sometimes we need to step back and look at the whole woman.

Herbal remedies have been studied in menopause with mixed results. Often this is because we are applying Western scientific theory where it may not totally relate. In the US we do not have the same certifications and regulation of herbal medicine as in other parts of the world, or herbal medicine practitioners. Herbs are "natural"; however, that is not necessarily synonymous with "safe." Using a reference such as this, written by an expert in medical herbalism, is key if you are going to explore using herbal medicine.

In this book, traditional herbal remedies and lifestyle interventions predominate. This is intentional. Hormone therapy has a role for some women and can be a huge benefit to those who need it. It is also a safe and beneficial intervention when used properly. But the cornerstone of menopause management is living a healthy lifestyle.

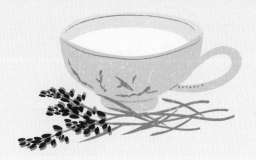

The key parts of this book, in my mind, are the nutrition, exercise, and mental wellness chapters, which present the ideal interventions a woman can take. This is the foundation of a long and healthy life after menopause and can moderate some of the age-related diseases that can impact quality of life.

Do not feel that if you cannot make all of the changes, you shouldn't make any. Pick one area to focus on and try to improve your behavior there. The most important advice I have here is to give yourself grace. You will not be perfect, but you can feel better if you improve your diet or exercise even 20 percent. And once you see some benefit, that will be inspiration to make more healthy changes.

This book presents you with the information you need. Approaching menopause from a place of knowledge and strength rather than fear and hype is key. Every woman needs a different cocktail of remedies, solutions, patience, and hope going into and through this process and transition. On the other side of the divide is a confidence and strength that is well worth it.

As women, we need more tools like this to help us live our best menopause in the second half of life.

Rebecca Dunsmoor-Su
MD MSCE NCMP

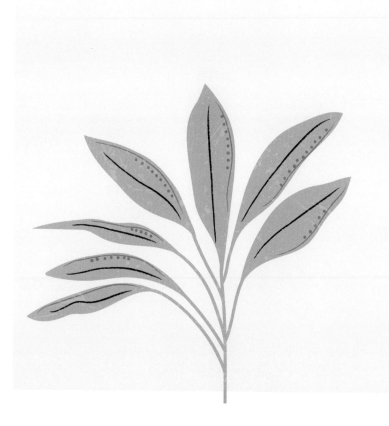

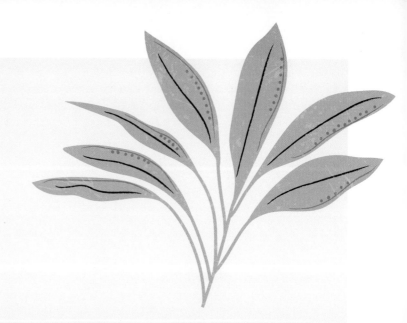

A NATURAL
MENOPAUSE

INTRODUCTION

Menopause is a time of great change, not only biologically but also physically and emotionally. Understanding what is happening to your body, and why, is key to introducing changes to your lifestyle and health to make the transition through menopause to the next stage of your life as smooth as possible.

All women will go through menopause at some point, which is defined as "the end of monthly cycles" from the Greek for "pause" and "cycle." At menopause the ovarian production of estrogen and progesterone falls significantly, as does testosterone, but to a lesser extent. It is generally accepted that you have gone through menopause when you have not had a period for a year, although this is not a definitive diagnosis. In reality, the physiology is far more complex. Your body undergoes a wide range of changes over many years—a decade or more—before you become post-menopausal.

The average age for a woman to go through menopause is 51.7 years, but perimenopause can start more than a decade earlier. Many women therefore begin to experience menopausal symptoms in their early to mid-40s, but fail to realize these changes are the start of menopause because they incorrectly believe they are too young or their symptoms are due to other issues.

Some women will also go through a premature menopause before the age of 40,

which may be due to genetic factors, surgery to remove the ovaries, or other treatments affecting ovarian function. See also page 12.

WHY MENOPAUSE HAPPENS

Each woman is born with a finite number of follicles, or egg sacs, in the ovaries in which mature eggs will develop. Although you are born with around 300,000 primordial follicles, other than the ones that result in ovulation, the remainder will naturally atrophy over the course of your life.

From puberty, the ovaries release an egg each month as part of your menstrual cycle, as well as producing key hormones such as estrogen, progesterone, and testosterone. No new follicles develop after birth, so by your 40s the number of eggs has declined significantly. At this point, the ovaries become more resistant to the hormones released from the pituitary gland, specifically follicle stimulating hormone (FSH) and luteinizing hormone (LH), and the monthly pattern of ovulation gradually declines along with the levels of key hormones.

" "

Menopause is the ideal time to focus on you, and the benefits that
natural remedies, exercise, mental wellness practices, nutrition, or HRT
can bring to your physical, mental, and spiritual well-being.

The menopause transition can extend over many years, and although it varies from woman to woman, it can be broken down into three main stages: perimenopause, menopause, and post-menopause.

PERIMENOPAUSE
Perimenopause is the time leading up to menopause when your body, ovarian function, and hormone levels undergo

seismic shifts. You may find that your periods alter, becoming more frequent and heavier, or more irregular and lighter. Because every woman is different, her menstrual cycle will change in a variable and unpredictable way, although genetic influence is a key factor.

You may not realize that you are perimenopausal and that your hormone levels are declining until you experience

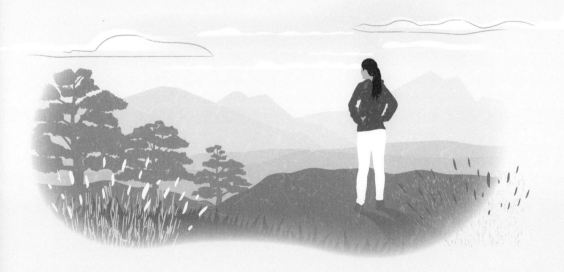

menopausal symptoms, usually vasomotor issues (hot flashes and night sweats) and insomnia initially. Many women are also aware of worsening PMS during the lead-up to menopause, and psychological problems such as heightened anxiety. See also pages 14–15.

MENOPAUSE

The main change you will notice at menopause is that your periods cease and conception will no longer be possible. In the lead-up to this, your menstrual cycle will usually become more unpredictable over several years before finally stopping.

POST-MENOPAUSE

Technically you are post-menopausal when you have not had a period for a year over the age of 50, and for two years under the age of 50, although this is not always the case.

Although some women find their symptoms ease after their periods stop, this is certainly not the norm, and studies show that a significant proportion of women will continue to experience serious problems for many years (on average five to seven years), although as many as 10–15 percent of women will still be suffering from symptoms more than a decade later.

It can be helpful for women to try to embrace these issues as the body settles into the "new normal," as well as seeking supportive measures to help cope with this challenging period of life. The next phase of life can be empowering if you manage it effectively.

PREMATURE AND EARLY MENOPAUSE

Premature menopause or premature ovarian insufficiency is when menopause happens before the age of 40, while an early menopause occurs before 45.

Around one percent of women will experience premature menopause, which is caused by a number of factors. It can be hereditary, so if your mother or grandmother had an early menopause, you may, too.

A premature or early menopause may be the result of surgical removal of your ovaries, most commonly due to benign conditions such as endometriosis, or more rarely due to cancer, where treatment may also involve radiotherapy and chemotherapy.

If you experience a premature or early menopause, it is highly recommended that you take HRT until at least the normal menopausal age of 51.7 to minimize menopausal symptoms as well as the risk of longer-term health problems, including osteoporosis and cardiovascular disease. See also Chapter 6.

However, if you have gone through an earlier menopause due to treatment for a hormone-responsive cancer (breast, endometrial, or ovarian), then HRT may be contraindicated and may not be recommended. See also Chapter 6.

WHY HORMONES ARE SO IMPORTANT

Fluctuation in hormone levels, in particular declining estrogen, causes many of the symptoms associated with menopause, as well as longer-term health issues that can arise later in life. Fortunately, there are many ways to counter the effects of these hormonal changes, including targeted exercise, optimal nutrition, herbal remedies, and stress management, as well as a wide range of hormone therapies. See also the Symptom Checker on pages 22–33.

Estrogen affects virtually every organ in the body including the brain, musculo-skeletal system (bones and joints), cardiovascular system (heart and lungs), urogenital system (bladder, uterus, and vagina), as well as skin, nails, and hair.

Estrogen also plays a key role in maintaining healthy bone density, and the decline in estrogen around menopause can be associated with a reduction in bone density, leading to osteopenia and, in more severe cases, osteoporosis.

Estrogen has a cardio-protective effect on the heart and vascular system, and is the main reason why women are less likely to experience heart disease than men. When estrogen levels decline after menopause, however, there is a relatively rapid rise in the incidence of cardiovascular disease, which is a key contributor to female morbidity and mortality in later years.

Awareness of these risks allows you to look at lifestyle and health changes to maximize bone density and protect your heart, including exercise (see Chapter 5) and good nutrition (see Chapter 4).

THE KEY HORMONES

ESTROGEN

The primary female sex hormone, estrogen, stimulates breast growth during puberty and maintains the menstrual cycle. Estrogen helps regulate mood and is important for heart and bone health.

PROGESTERONE

Progesterone is an important hormone during pregnancy and also plays a role in the menstrual cycle by stimulating the uterine lining to shed each month.

TESTOSTERONE

Traditionally viewed as the "male" hormone, testosterone regulates sex drive and can aid sleep, mood, and energy levels. It also helps maintain muscle tone.

Estrogen also helps regulate serotonin levels in the brain, and modifies the production of endorphins: both of these are "feel-good" transmitters in the brain. This key link explains the frequent association between low mood and heightened anxiety, which all are too often associated with menopause. Understanding that these psychological issues are largely unavoidable and are directly due to fluctuating hormone levels enables you to make positive changes to improve your mental well-being, including targeted exercise such as yoga, and breathing and relaxation techniques. See also Chapters 3 and 5.

RECOGNIZING THE SIGNS

While most women are aware of the more common menopausal symptoms such as mood swings and hot flashes, there are in fact over 30 recognized symptoms of menopause, from dry eyes and poor memory to bloating, heart palpitations, and brittle nails. Most women will experience many of the symptoms, and it is rare for a woman to go through menopause without encountering any at all.

Many early symptoms may be quite subtle, and women are often unaware that they are experiencing the start of perimenopause. Initial symptoms may include thinning hair or temporary lapses in short-term memory, and other classic symptoms tend to follow with time. For some women, symptoms gradually lessen in the years after menopause, but in many cases women can continue to suffer long after their periods have ceased: in this group HRT may be the only way to address the protracted symptoms. See also Chapter 6.

KNOWLEDGE IS KEY

Menopausal symptoms can vary considerably between individual women and will also change as the menopause transition progresses. Awareness of the wide range of menopausal symptoms is absolutely key, as is the knowledge that you may experience one or more symptoms at different stages (see diagram, right) and that there is a

" "

Understanding why you are experiencing changes during menopause, looking out for possible symptom triggers, and making positive changes to your lifestyle can help smooth your path through menopause.

SIGNS YOU MAY BE MENOPAUSAL

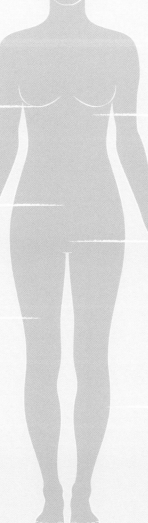

- Hair thinning, loss, and dryness
- Tinnitus
- Dry eyes
- Altered sense of smell
- Acne
- Facial hair
- Wrinkles and dry skin
- Dry or burning mouth
- Gum problems

- Sore breasts
- Change in body odor/ excessive sweating

- Digestive problems and abdominal bloating
- Constipation
- Weight gain

- Increased allergies
- Restless leg syndrome
- Itchy skin
- Prickling and tingling sensation on skin
- Brittle nails

- Mood swings
- Depression
- Irritability
- Anxiety and panic attacks
- Brain fog and memory lapses
- Difficulty concentrating
- Disrupted sleep and fatigue
- Dizzy spells
- Headaches and migraines

- Hot flashes/heat intolerance
- Night sweats
- Irregular heartbeat or palpitations

- Irregular and/or heavy periods
- Stress incontinence
- Loss of libido
- Recurrent urinary tract infections
- Vaginal dryness and soreness

- Stiff and aching joints and muscles

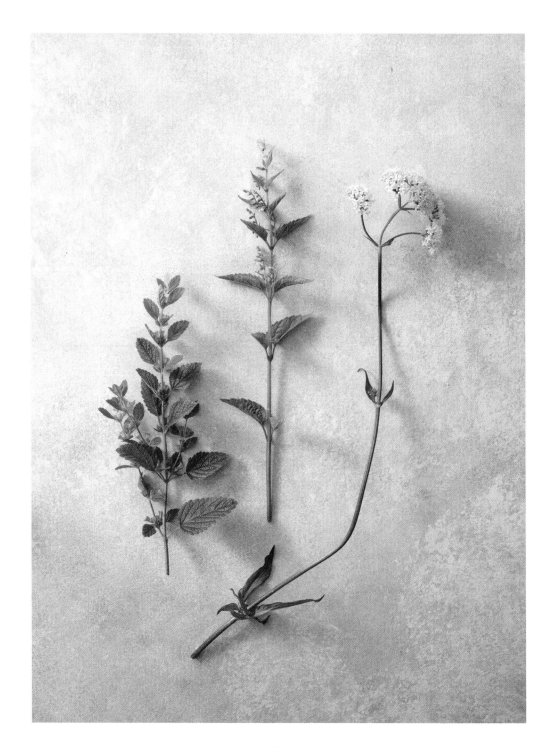

physiological explanation for your anxious feelings, low mood, aches and pains, or dry eyes can be very reassuring. With knowledge comes power, and once you are aware that the symptoms are due to menopause, seeking help will be easier.

A NATURAL APPROACH

Although menopause is a time of great change, it is also a perfect opportunity to assess your life and explore new avenues to maximize your health and mental well-being, both during and after menopause.

Whether you amend your exercise routine or diet, take supplements or herbal remedies, or adopt mental wellness practices, there are a number of ways that you can ensure your transition is as smooth as possible and you are physically and mentally ready for the next stage of your life. You can also do all of the above while taking HRT.

FOCUS ON THE POSITIVES

Focus on cutting out anything detrimental to your well-being, whether this is unhelpful thoughts or unhealthy elements in your diet. Try to eliminate adverse triggers such as alcohol, stress, or caffeine, which frequently exacerbate symptoms such as hot flashes and insomnia. Instead look at swapping in herbal teas that can relax and aid sleep (see Chapter 2), or use CBT (see pages 112–119) to calm the body and mind and eliminate stress, promoting mental well-being.

Instead of feeling stressed or negative about your body or future, look at ways to calm, energize, or concentrate your mind, such as an aromatherapy massage (see Chapter 2), yoga (see pages 186–197), or mental wellness exercises (see Chapter 3).

Try to live as mindfully as possible, focus on the positives in your life, however large or small they may be, and set aside time for yourself. This will help decrease stress levels and reduce feelings of anxiety you may be experiencing.

BENEFITS FOR LONG-TERM HEALTH

Introducing lifestyle changes around the time of menopause can not only help relieve troublesome symptoms, but will also have long-lasting health benefits into old age. Knowledge and awareness of the impact that declining hormone levels have on your body means you can be proactive and explore different ways to maximize your health, for example, increasing your intake of brain-friendly foods, using herbal remedies to improve sleep, or simply enjoying regular yoga to maintain flexibility and tone.

Maintaining bone density is of the utmost importance, both during and after menopause. Although bone mass and density will naturally decline, you can focus on strengthening exercises (see Chapter 5) and good nutrition (see Chapter 4), both of which help maintain bone health.

Cardiovascular disease can be a major concern around menopause, so making sure you reduce stress levels (see Chapter 3), follow a heart-friendly diet (see Chapter 4), and exercise effectively (see Chapter 5) will help keep your heart in good shape.

ADOPTING A HOLISTIC APPROACH

Many women find that the best way to maintain optimum health during menopause is to use a combination of approaches. For example, you may find that reducing triggers such as alcohol or stress, practicing CBT, or taking herbal remedies will reduce hot flashes; while a combination of journaling, yoga, and aromatherapy will reduce anxiety and keep you calm and focused. By improving aspects of your diet and by exercising more, you may find that your overall health improves and your mood is boosted, too. Try out different approaches to see what suits you best, and remember none of the approaches in this book is exclusive, and all can be used alongside HRT.

- **Herbal remedies** can confer a wealth of benefits during menopause. Some herbal remedies will help with hormonal balance, while other herbal remedies can aid digestive health and liver function, which are vital for hormone manufacture and breakdown. Some herbal remedies can help reduce inflammation, while others will support well-being by improving sleep quality, boosting mood, or calming anxious feelings.

Herbal remedies act on many systems in the body, including the nervous and hormonal systems, and thus not only improve many menopausal symptoms but, by addressing the root cause of the symptoms, they can also provide a general tonic that improves overall health and well-being. See also Chapter 2.

- **Aromatherapy and massage** are key for self-care and for connecting with your body. They can not only help you to accept the changes your body is going through, but also appreciate everything it does for you and maintain your feelings of self-worth. They can also assist with relaxation and reenergizing, as well as improving mood and relieving various menopausal symptoms including anxiety, itchy/dry skin, and loss of libido. See also Chapter 2.

- **Mental wellness practices** can help you figure out why you are feeling the way you do and how best to approach and prepare for this time of physical and mental transition. For some women, mindfulness, journaling, CBT, or visualization will help maintain a positive outlook and calm feelings of anxiety. For other women, seeking support from friends or family or seeing a menopause counselor may be the most beneficial approach.

Being able to do something positive can help you ground yourself, maintain calm, improve mood and sleep patterns, and generally have a more positive outlook

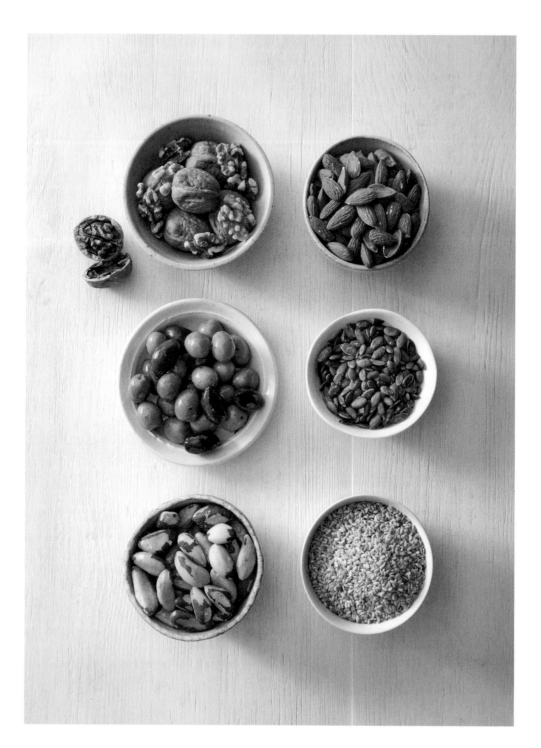

on life. Taking time to rest and reflect and to visualize what you want your future to look like can help you focus on changes you need to make and how best to move forward. See also Chapter 3.

- **Good nutrition and a well-balanced diet** will ensure that your body has everything it needs to adjust to the hormonal changes of menopause and maintain good overall health, as well as helping minimize some menopausal symptoms. A well-balanced diet can help you maintain bone density, as well as a healthy heart, gut, liver, and brain. It can also help with weight management, which is beneficial because weight gain is a common issue for many menopausal women.

Because many women who enter perimenopause or menopause are deficient in key nutrients, this is a productive time to look at what you are eating, how you can improve aspects of your diet, what you should be cutting back on, and whether you should be taking any supplements. See also Chapter 4.

- **Exercise is important** throughout your life, but is absolutely vital at menopause and beyond. Regular exercise will not only help maintain bone density, aid weight management, and decrease your risk of cardiovascular disease, but is also proven to significantly boost mental health and general well-being.

There are so many different types of exercise available that, regardless of your fitness level or experience, you will be able to find something you enjoy, such as brisk walking, swimming, or yoga. Weight-bearing exercise is particularly beneficial at menopause to maintain bone and muscle mass, and there are specially designed programs on pages 162–185 to help you get started or amend your existing exercise regimen. See also Chapter 5.

- **Modern HRT** is arguably the most effective way to reduce the severity of all physical and psychological symptoms associated with menopause and can be life-changing for many women. HRT can also provide major longer-term health benefits—in particular for your skeleton, cardiovascular system, and brain—which can not only extend your lifespan but also ensure that you enjoy a far better quality of life. It is important to stress that it is safe to take HRT alongside all the natural approaches outlined in this book. See also Chapter 6.

HOW TO USE THIS BOOK

Use each chapter to help you navigate the menopause transition in your own unique way. Embark on your personal journey with all the information you need to make informed choices about how best to prepare your body physically, mentally, and spiritually for menopause and life going forward. Adapt your existing wellness routines or embrace new ones, whether or not you are taking HRT, so that you can make the next stage in your wellness journey a healthy, joyful, and positive one.

A HOLISTIC APPROACH TO OPTIMUM HEALTH

HERBAL REMEDIES

Exploring herbal remedies can help you manage menopausal concerns, as well as address the root causes of symptoms and enhance overall wellness (see Chapter 2).

AROMATHERAPY

Essential oils and massage can be very beneficial for both physical and emotional well-being. Different oils can help calm, boost mood, aid sleep, or invigorate (see Chapter 2).

MENTAL WELLNESS

Techniques such as mindfulness, visualization, and CBT can be very useful tools if you are finding the menopause transition unsettling or difficult (see Chapter 3).

GOOD NUTRITION

The Menopause Diet can help protect your heart, bones, and brain. It can also help regulate your weight and relieve menopausal symptoms (see Chapter 4).

EXERCISE

The best way to maintain good health and fitness, and protect your bones and heart, is through regular weight-bearing exercises. Yoga is also key for maintaining mobility and calm (see Chapter 5).

HRT

HRT can reduce or prevent many symptoms of menopause as well as helping maintain good general health, in particular bone density and cardiovascular health (see Chapter 6).

Supporting your body throughout menopause can confer long-lasting health benefits to your bones, heart, gut, and brain, as well as improving your mood and overall mental well-being.

SYMPTOM CHECKER

While some women experience very few symptoms during perimenopause and menopause, for many the dramatic hormonal changes during this time are associated with a wide range of unwanted and often debilitating symptoms, from hot flashes and aching joints to anxiety and loss of libido. Fortunately, there are ways to minimize or even prevent these problems.

Recognizing that the adverse symptoms you are experiencing are quite normal and are due to changing hormone levels associated with perimenopause and menopause will help you address these problems effectively by finding ways to transition smoothly—and with positivity—to the next phase of your life.

WHAT TO EXPECT

Every woman's experience of menopause is individual, and as you go through perimenopause and menopause you are likely to encounter various symptoms at different stages of the pathway and, in some cases, even well beyond menopause itself.

While some symptoms can be very obvious, such as hot flashes or menopausal acne, others may be less evident, including psychological issues such as low mood and anxiety.

HOW TO USE THE SYMPTOM CHECKER

On the following pages you will find the most common menopausal symptoms and a range of approaches you can take in order to minimize their effects. Whether you have aching joints, night sweats, or mood swings, there are suggestions for how you can address the problems. By changing your diet or exercise regimen, using essential oils, practicing mindfulness, taking HRT, or investigating herbal remedies, you can try to minimize or even stop the symptoms.

HOT FLASHES AND NIGHT SWEATS

Hot flashes and night sweats, which are called vasomotor symptoms, are the commonest menopausal symptoms of all and affect more than 90 percent of women, impacting on the body's thermoregulatory control center in the brain. Women can experience a variety of symptoms including a rushing sensation of heat, facial flushing, uncontrollable sweating, and palpitations. Night sweats can lead to significant sleep disruption and chronic fatigue.

WHAT YOU CAN DO
There are a number of ways to reduce vasomotor symptoms, including avoiding triggers and taking herbal remedies.

Herbal Remedies
- Red clover (see page 64) and black cohosh (see page 61) have been found to be effective in reducing hot flashes.

Aromatherapy
- Use essential oils such as sweet fennel (see page 72), cypress (see page 75), or clary sage (see page 69) in a spritz, diffuser, or inhaler.

Mental Wellness
- When you feel a flash starting, do not be embarrassed. Focus on a breathing exercise to reduce the intensity (see pages 91–3).
- Use CBT techniques to minimize the effects of the hot flash (see page 116).

Nutrition
- Eat plenty of omega-3 fatty acids found in oily fish and flaxseeds (see page 132) or take an omega-3 supplement (see pages 150–51).
- Eat foods rich in hormone-balancing phytoestrogens such as soy, tofu, chickpeas, and lentils (see page 149).
- Cut back or avoid triggers such as hot drinks, alcohol, and caffeinated drinks.

Exercise
- Many women report a reduction in the frequency and severity of hot flashes when they exercise regularly (see Chapter 5).

HRT
- Taking HRT effectively reduces both the frequency and severity of hot flashes and night sweats, often within a few weeks of commencing treatment (see Chapter 6).

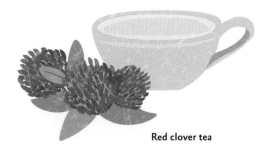

Red clover tea

MOOD SWINGS

Changes in mood are extremely common during menopause. Many women feel their emotions become erratic and uncontrollable: they may feel low much of the time; or fine one moment, then suddenly irritable and tearful the next. These feelings can be very confusing and upsetting, affecting self-confidence and relationships.

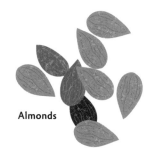

Almonds

WHAT YOU CAN DO

You can address mood swings by taking herbal remedies, eating mood-boosting foods, and talking about your concerns.

Herbal Remedies

- Drink relaxing herbal teas on a daily basis. Try skullcap (see page 51), oat straw (see page 54), lemon balm (see page 45), valerian (see page 53), or St. John's wort (see page 48).

Aromatherapy

- Choose essential oils that are a tonic for conflicting emotions—try geranium (see page 71), frankincense, or bergamot (see page 74).

Mental Wellness

- Take one minute to be mindful to help you accept things as they are (see page 94).
- Focus on a breathing exercise to reconnect with your rational brain (see pages 91–3).
- Don't bottle up your feelings—talk to friends, family, or a counselor about how you are feeling (see pages 83–5).
- Incorporate relaxation techniques into your routine to help you de-stress (see Chapter 3).

- Use CBT techniques to calm and balance emotions (see page 114).

Nutrition

- Ensure your diet is rich in hormone-balancing phytoestrogens such as chickpeas, soy products, and lentils (see page 149).
- Eat foods rich in magnesium such as almonds or Brazil nuts (see page 144), or take a magnesium supplement (see pages 150–51).
- Eat mood-boosting foods that are high in omega-3 fatty acids (see page 132) or take an omega-3 supplement (see pages 150–51).
- Eat regularly to maintain consistent blood-sugar levels (see Chapter 4).

Exercise

- Exercise promotes the release of mood-boosting endorphins in your body, and regular exercise is correlated to improvements in mood (see Chapter 5).

HRT

- HRT can improve low mood and mood swings because it works on the estrogen receptors located in the brain (see Chapter 6).

ANXIETY

During menopause, adrenaline and cortisol are released as the body tries to rebalance itself while estrogen and progesterone levels gradually decrease. This can cause mood swings (see opposite) as well as heightened anxiety, which is often associated with heart palpitations during perimenopause. Anxious feelings can also be exacerbated by insomnia (see page 26), creating a vicious cycle where minor worries become magnified.

WHAT YOU CAN DO

Don't bottle up your worries. Talk to someone about them and try relaxation techniques such as yoga and mindfulness.

Herbal Remedies
- Try herbal teas, in particular lavender (see page 47), lemon balm (see page 45), or skullcap (see page 51). Drink them hot or chilled with apple juice and slices of fruit.

Aromatherapy
- Geranium (see page 71), rose (see page 77), bergamot (see page 74), and cypress (see page 75) essential oils can all help relieve anxiety.

Mental Wellness
- Write in your worry journal every day to relieve anxiety (see page 104).
- Put down your phone and switch off from negative technology (see page 98).

Nutrition
- Eat foods rich in magnesium and potassium such as bananas, quinoa, avocado, raspberries, nuts, seeds, and legumes (see page 144).

- Avoid caffeine in all forms (see page 130).
- Boost your intake of vitamin D—spend enough time in the sunshine and eat foods rich in vitamin D (see page 141) or take a vitamin D supplement (see page 150).

Exercise
- Exercise can boost mood, improve sleep, and heighten self-esteem, which together can reduce anxiety (see Chapter 5).
- Yoga can help relax you and calm your mind (see pages 186–197).

HRT
- HRT can help relieve anxiety and promote a calmer mindset (see Chapter 6).

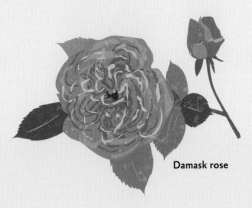

Damask rose

FATIGUE AND INSOMNIA

Insomnia is a common problem during menopause. Many women find that they struggle to go to sleep or wake up in the early hours of the morning and can't go back to sleep again. In addition, many women are woken by night sweats, which further disrupt sleep. When sleepless nights persist for months, or even years, the result can be extremely debilitating, adversely affecting energy levels, clarity, and focus, as well as mental health.

WHAT YOU CAN DO

Herbal remedies and essential oils can be very effective. Also try relaxation practices and yoga to aid better sleep.

Herbal Remedies

- Support yourself throughout the day with a teaspoon of revitalizing maca powder (see page 65) at breakfast; a licorice and mint tea (see page 56) when you're fading; and calming herbs such as chamomile (see page 49) or lavender (see page 47) at night.

Aromatherapy

- Use bergamot (see page 74) or lavender essential oils to calm your nervous system.

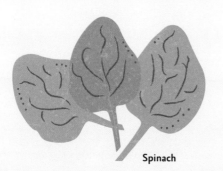

Spinach

Mental Wellness

- Practice color breathing (see page 92).
- Deeply relax every part of your body by doing a body scan (see page 102).
- Use CBT techniques to help you sleep better (see page 118).

Nutrition

- Eat foods high in iron such as spinach and lentils, plus plenty of high-quality protein (see page 135) to provide energy and minimize feelings of fatigue.
- Avoid caffeine, especially in the afternoon, to help with sleep.

Exercise

- Research suggests that exercise may reduce insomnia by decreasing anxiety and helping regulate your body clock (see Chapter 5).
- Practice yoga to relax and ready your body and mind for sleep (see pages 186–197).

HRT

- Rebalancing hormones through HRT can aid sleep and thus boost energy levels and reduce feelings of fatigue (see Chapter 6)..

BRAIN FOG

Menopausal women can struggle to remember simple tasks and concentrate fully. This can be both frustrating and distressing and can significantly impact many aspects of life. These symptoms are a physiological response to the depletion of estrogen, which triggers hormone receptors in the brain responsible for clarity.

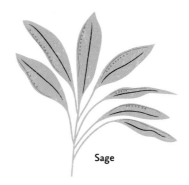

Sage

WHAT YOU CAN DO

Recognize that it is normal that your memory may be temporarily affected and don't panic. Increase your intake of brain-boosting foods.

Herbal Remedies

- Have a morning cup of rosemary (see page 55), licorice (see page 56), and sage (see page 62) herbal tea to help lift brain fog.

Aromatherapy

- Use bergamot (see page 74) essential oil in an inhaler or diffuser to help with clarity.

Mental Wellness

- Take regular breaks away from the task at hand to give you the opportunity to think clearly and rationally.
- Take a mindful walk (see page 96) when you feel as if your brain needs a break.
- Keep a to-do list but with a maximum of three things on it so it isn't overwhelming.

Nutrition

- Boost your intake of vitamin B12 through foods including eggs, liver, salmon, and sardines (see page 140) or take a B vitamin supplement (see page 150) to help improve brain clarity and memory.
- Eat foods rich in omega-3 fatty acids such as salmon and sardines (see page 132) or take an omega-3 supplement (see pages 150–51).
- Increase your intake of antioxidant-rich foods such as citrus fruits, green leafy vegetables, avocado, and turmeric to help protect your brain.

Exercise

- Exercise releases chemicals in your body that can sharpen your focus and help you to concentrate. Research also suggests that exercise can improve memory and slow down cognitive decline as you age (see Chapter 5).

HRT

- HRT can result in substantial improvements in mental clarity, memory, and concentration by boosting declining hormone levels (see Chapter 6).

JOINT PAIN AND MUSCLE STIFFNESS

Many women find that their joints start to ache and feel generally stiff during menopause, especially first thing in the morning. This is a result of the gradual reduction in estrogen levels, as the hormone is critical for good bone and joint health throughout the body.

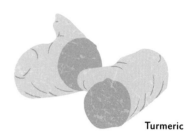

Turmeric

WHAT YOU CAN DO

Exercise, a good diet, and staying hydrated are key to maintaining bone and muscle strength, which helps with mobility and suppleness.

Herbal Remedies

■ Depending on the underlying problems, the following herbs may help: licorice (see page 56), black cohosh (see page 61), chamomile (see page 49), red clover (see page 64), or dandelion root (see page 67).

Aromatherapy

■ Use a compress or massage oil made from one or a blend of the following essential oils: cypress (see page 75), clary sage (see page 69), rosemary, lavender, or lemongrass.

Mental Wellness

■ Work through a body scan practice (see page 102) to relax joints and muscles.

Nutrition

■ Eat omega-3 anti-inflammatory foods such as oily fish regularly (see page 132) or take an omega-3 supplement (see pages 150–51).

■ Add turmeric, ginger, cinnamon, and garlic to food when you are cooking as they will naturally help reduce inflammation.

■ Make sure your diet is rich in whole, unprocessed foods and fresh fruit and vegetables (see Chapter 4).

■ Drink plenty of water to keep tissues moist and supple (see page 137), and limit your alcohol consumption.

■ Eat foods that are rich in magnesium such as almonds and spinach (see page 144) or take a magnesium supplement (see pages 150–51).

Exercise

■ Yoga and stretching can improve mobility and flexibility, which helps reduce joint pain (see pages 186–197).

■ Strength training strengthens muscles, ligaments, and the tendons surrounding joints, helping alleviate joint pain and generally keep you supple (see Chapter 5).

HRT

■ Many women find HRT helps alleviate joint symptoms, reducing discomfort and improving mobility (see Chapter 6).

UROGENITAL PROBLEMS

Declining estrogen levels are responsible for many urogenital problems that commonly arise during menopause. A lack of estrogen affects the lining of both the vagina and bladder, causing these tissues to become thinner and more sensitive. This results in an increased susceptibility to problems such as vaginal discomfort and urinary tract infections. These changes are jointly known as genitourinary syndrome of menopause.

WHAT YOU CAN DO

Good hydration is essential, but you may also find relief from herbal remedies. Localized HRT is also very effective.

Herbal Remedies

- Drink a daily cup or two of chamomile (see page 49), marigold (see page 59), or red clover (see page 64) herbal teas.

Mental Wellness

- Talk to someone—don't let embarrassment stop you from getting the help and support you need (see Chapter 3).

Nutrition

- Drink unsweetened cranberry juice, which can be beneficial for UTIs because cranberries stop bacteria from attaching to the walls of the urinary tract.
- Drink plenty of water (see page 137); not drinking enough will cause your urine to be more concentrated, which can irritate the bladder and lead to UTIs.

- Cut back on caffeine because it can irritate the bladder further.

Exercise

- Yoga (see page 186–197), swimming, strength training, and Pilates can help strengthen the core and pelvic muscles, which may relieve pelvic pain (see Chapter 5).

HRT

- Because HRT boosts estrogen levels, it is beneficial for bladder, vaginal, and pelvic concerns.
- Local HRT pessaries or cream can also effectively target specific urogenital problems (see Chapter 6).

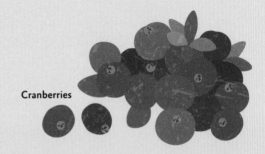

Cranberries

WEIGHT GAIN

Women often struggle with their weight and body shape as they go through menopause. Fat tends to accumulate around the abdomen, resulting in classic "middle-age spread." These changes partly occur due to loss of muscle mass (sarcopenia), which gradually declines with age, as well as the reduction in metabolic rate. As weight gain can have an adverse effect on health, mood, self-esteem, and libido, it is vital to address it effectively.

WHAT YOU CAN DO

A combination of good nutrition and regular exercise is the best way to make sure that you have a calorie deficit and don't put on weight.

Herbal Remedies

- Try drinking sage (see page 62) or rosemary (see page 55) tea each morning.

Aromatherapy

- Use essential oils that can help alleviate bloating, such as cypress (see page 75).

Mental Wellness

- If weight gain is concerning you, seek support by talking to a registered professional who can help (see Chapter 3).

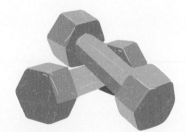

Weights for strength training

Nutrition

- Eat wholesome, unprocessed foods that are high in fiber (see page 138).
- Downsize your portions, keep a food diary, and cook from scratch at home. Limit high-calorie intake, eliminate junk food, and avoid high-fat takeout (see Chapter 4).
- Improve your gut microbiome by taking prebiotics and probiotics (see page 146).

Exercise

- Exercise boosts energy expenditure and can help you maintain a calorie deficit if you want to lose weight (see Chapter 5).
- When dieting, strength training can help you lose fat while also preserving muscle mass.

HRT

- HRT has a direct impact on weight because it helps maintain muscle mass and metabolic rate, and may also boost declining energy levels and improve motivation, meaning you are more likely to focus successfully on healthy eating, exercise, and other weight-loss measures (see Chapter 6).

DIGESTIVE ISSUES

Fluctuating hormone levels affect every part of the body, including the digestive tract. Menopausal women commonly find that their gut health suffers, resulting in problems such as abdominal bloating, fluid retention, and constipation. Conditions such as IBS may also worsen, exacerbating symptoms such as abdominal pain and bowel problems.

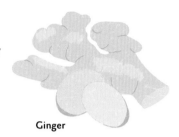

Ginger

WHAT YOU CAN DO

Maintaining good gut health through a healthy diet is key, while natural remedies are often effective at helping with symptoms.

Herbal Remedies

- Ease digestion by incorporating herbal teas such as chamomile (see page 49), lemon balm (see page 45), lavender (see page 47), valerian (see page 53), and dandelion root (see page 67) into your daily fluid intake.

Aromatherapy

- Massage your abdomen using a massage oil made with one or more of the following essential oils: sweet fennel (see page 72), clary sage (see page 69), or sweet orange.

Mental Wellness

- Stress and anxiety can affect digestion, so practice calming breathing exercises (see pages 91–3).

Nutrition

- Use ginger in cooking; it helps reduce bloating and other digestive issues.

- Boost your intake of fiber (see page 138). For example, include chia seeds in your diet.
- Eat plenty of whole grains to support healthy digestion by reducing constipation and feeding healthy gut bacteria.
- Eat fermented foods such as yogurt, kefir, and sauerkraut to feed good gut bacteria. These contain probiotics (see also page 146), which can aid digestion.
- The gelatin found in bone broth can help improve digestion and protect your intestinal wall. It may also be useful in improving inflammatory bowel conditions.

Exercise

- Moderate exercise increases blood flow to the digestive tract, which can help achieve more efficient digestion (see Chapter 5).
- Moderate exercise may help alleviate bloating, stomach cramps, and constipation.

HRT

- The hormones found in HRT directly impact gut function, particularly motility, and can help relieve many common digestive problems (see Chapter 6).

LOSS OF LIBIDO

Loss of libido (sex drive) during and beyond menopause is a very common issue. Libido in women is very complex and can be affected by numerous factors including low energy levels, lack of sleep, low mood, anxiety, and poor self-esteem. In addition, some women experience localized problems such as vaginal dryness.

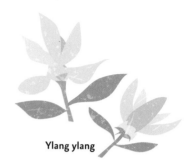

Ylang ylang

WHAT YOU CAN DO

Loss of libido can often be helped with natural remedies or HRT, but boosting mood through nutrition and exercise is also key.

Herbal Remedies

- Chaste tree (see page 60) may help revitalize your libido, but it does need to be taken for several months to be effective.
- Address energy levels by adding maca powder (see page 65) to your breakfast.

Aromatherapy

- Use rose (see page 77), clary sage (see page 69), or ylang ylang essential oils.

Mental Wellness

- Talk to your partner or a doctor or therapist if loss of libido is a concern for you. Don't suffer in silence (see Chapter 3).

Nutrition

- Make sure your diet is high in antioxidant-rich foods such as walnuts, lean meat, fish, green tea, and dark chocolate because they help increase circulation.

- Eat a diet high in hormone-balancing phytoestrogens such as flax seeds, chickpeas, and tofu (see page 149).
- Enjoy foods high in zinc such as oysters, crab, and pine nuts.
- Boost your intake of foods that contain plenty of vitamin C such as broccoli and oranges because they aid circulation. Or take a supplement (see page 150).

Exercise

- Cardiovascular exercise and strength training can boost mood and self-esteem, and can help you maintain a toned body, all of which can have a positive effect on libido (see Chapter 5).
- Yoga can help you relax and recharge (see pages 186–197).

HRT

- HRT can be extremely effective at improving libido and addressing local vaginal problems, including dryness and discomfort. Estrogen plays a role in this area, and local HRT can be of particular benefit (see Chapter 6).

SKIN AND HAIR CHANGES

Women frequently notice changes in their skin around the time of menopause, including loss of firmness and tone, an increase in fine lines and wrinkles, general dryness, and increased itching. Due to the delicate balance between estrogen and testosterone, some women may develop acne and increased facial hair. It is also not unusual for women to find their hair starts to thin and grow more slowly, with a loss of volume and shine.

WHAT YOU CAN DO

Regular moisturizing, staying hydrated, and eating foods that boost collagen production can all help with dry skin and wrinkles.

Herbal Remedies

- Take chaste tree (see page 60) every morning over several months for skin health.
- Drink marigold (see page 59), red clover (see page 64), sage (see page 62), or rosemary (see page 55) herbal teas to improve skin.

Aromatherapy

- Make a facial oil using geranium (see page 71) and rose (see page 77) essential oils.
- Use rosemary essential oil as a scalp tonic.

Mental Wellness

- Talk about changes you are experiencing and seek answers. It can be empowering to take back control (see Chapter 3).

Nutrition

- Enjoy oily fish a couple of times a week as they are high in omega-3 fatty acids (see page 132), which help keep your skin soft.

- Drink plenty of water every day to keep your skin hydrated (see page 137).
- Eat foods rich in vitamin E, which helps protect cells; and vitamin C, which is beneficial for maintaining skin tissue.

Exercise

- Many dermatologists believe that as exercise improves blood circulation it can help deliver oxygen and nutrients to your skin and hair follicles, promoting skin cell growth and preventing hair loss (see Chapter 5).

HRT

- HRT can boost skin texture and tone, reduce wrinkles, and resolve menopausal acne. It can also improve hair resilience and prevent nail thinning (see Chapter 6).

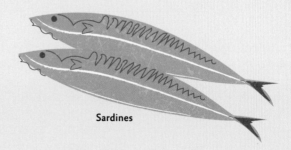

Sardines

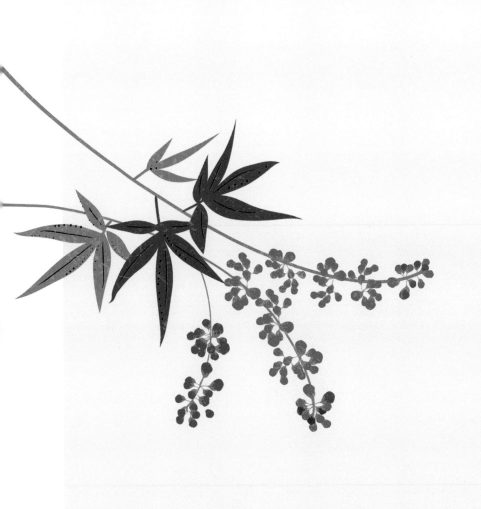

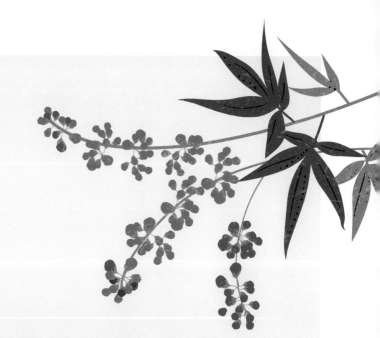

NATURAL REMEDIES

INTRODUCTION

Natural remedies offer women wide-reaching health benefits through a remarkably diverse range of healing, rejuvenating, and nutrient compounds. Herbal remedies and aromatherapy can help relieve many of the common symptoms of menopause, including hot flashes, insomnia, and anxiety.

The history of herbal medicine is ancient and can be seen in every culture on Earth. The most familiar of these are Ayurveda, Traditional Chinese Medicine (TCM), and Western Herbal Medicine. The World Health Organization estimates 70 percent of the world's population uses herbal medicine as a main system of medicine.

BENEFITS OF HERBAL REMEDIES

Herbal remedies are a specialized group of plants containing many compounds, including beneficial aromatic oils, which work together and can nourish and help your body function better. Your body often processes herbs as if they were food rather than drugs, despite the fact that plants contain compounds that have medicinal benefits. They can help improve your general health, meaning you are better able to adapt to changes that menopause brings.

Herbal remedies such as red clover (see page 64) can help with hormonal balance during menopause as they encourage beneficial estrogenlike compounds found naturally in your body after menopause. Other herbal remedies such as St. John's wort (see page 48) balance menopausal hormones by improving liver function and digestive health, which play an important role in hormone manufacture and breakdown.

Many herbal remedies have no direct effect on estrogen, but excel at reducing inflammation, while others such as sage (see page 62) help prevent recurrent infections, alleviating health problems that cause symptoms at menopause.

Herbal remedies can also provide numerous ways to support mental health and well-being, whether used internally as teas, tinctures, and capsules, or externally as whole herbs or aromatherapy oils that can uplift, soothe, and relax. Your hormones are not separate from your nervous system, so herbs and essential oils can provide mental restoration at menopause.

REDUCING MENOPAUSAL SYMPTOMS

There are many effective herbal remedies that can help ease hot flashes and night

" "

Changes during menopause can be a trigger for women
to rediscover themselves. Western herbal medicine emphasizes
an empathic approach, helping women redirect attention back
to their own well-being and the need for healing.

sweats, such as black cohosh (see page 61). Other herbal remedies such as valerian (see page 53) can help improve sleep, while oat straw (see page 54) and lemon balm (see page 45) are known to reduce anxiety and support your emotional health.

Herbs such as licorice (see page 56) and marigold (see page 59) can be used singly or in combination to ease skin soreness, dryness, or recurrent infections or inflammation that can be part of the menopausal landscape. When herbal remedies are applied to the root causes of your symptoms, the benefits can be long-lasting well beyond the end of treatment.

AN HERBAL APPROACH

Finding a practitioner with extensive knowledge of herbal remedies—whether a Naturopath, medical doctor, or functional medicine doctor—is important in order to assess your constitution, vitality, and phase before developing a comprehensive treatment plan and recommending individualized herbs.

Herbs are rarely prescribed in isolation, so even though lavender may help ease a headache, so might lemon balm, or passionflower, and a mixture of them all might be even more effective. Another woman may respond better to a blend of oat flowers, St. John's wort, and lemon balm.

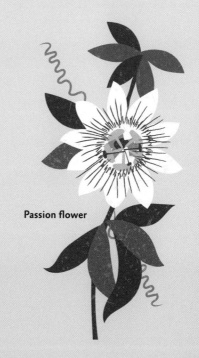

Passion flower

HERBAL REMEDIES VERSUS MEDICINES

Medicinal herbs may not be as strong as mono-chemicals (single chemicals, largely used by pharmaceuticals), but they contain many beneficial compounds, and due to their complexity have a broader therapeutic range and considerably fewer side effects.

Although there is a tendency to think about herbs from a modern medical viewpoint, which seeks single chemicals to address specific symptoms (for example, a painkiller for a headache), herbal medicine is much more successful when it is used to support the individual, optimizing inherent anti-inflammatory mechanisms. Herbal medicine is truly person-centered medicine, and although herbs have specific benefits (see box), success can also be attributed to all the other beneficial compounds found within the same plant.

HERBAL HELP FOR HORMONE CHANGE

Your body should manufacture a range of compounds with many of the benefits of estrogen after menopause, but different parts of the body need to work together to manufacture them. The liver, adrenal glands, gut, microbiome, and subcutaneous fat are all involved in hormone production,

WHAT MANY HERBAL REMEDIES CONTAIN

- Nutrients, including vitamins, minerals, and specific tissue tonics
- Antioxidants
- Anti-inflammatories
- Antibacterial and antiviral compounds
- Compounds that aid absorption of beneficial elements/restrict the absorption of less-beneficial ones.

modification, and elimination as a cycle. Postmenopausal hormone production therefore requires healthy function and communication among them all.

Gentle, relaxing herbs such as lemon balm (see page 45), valerian (see page 53), and skullcap (see page 51) can help ease stress that negatively affects hormone balance. Drinking herbal teas can also help you be mindful of staying hydrated, potentially reducing a reliance on alcohol to de-stress. Reducing the effects of stress takes the pressure off the immune system too, making you more able to face the challenges of adaptation at menopause, and helping create a positive cycle of self-care.

❝ ❞

Herbs are made up of many of the things that your body needs during menopause. They can help you optimize your well-being and flourish.

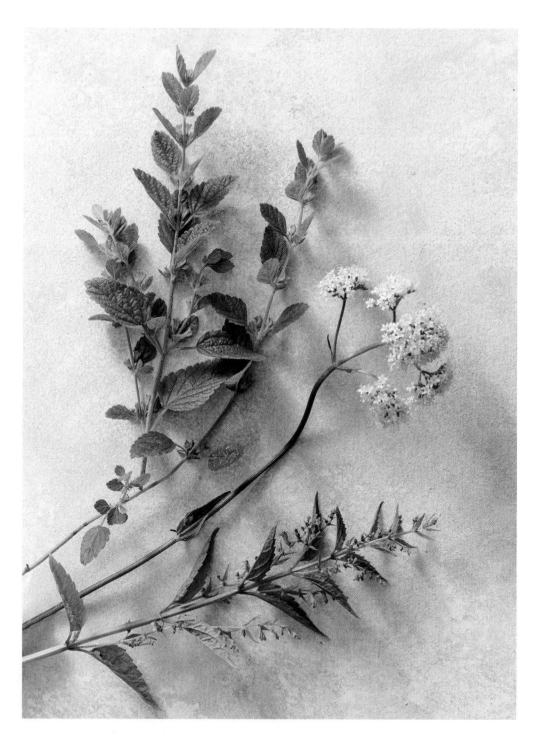

HERBAL REMEDIES VERSUS HRT

The study of medicinal plants has greatly increased our understanding of the hormone estrogen, and its role before and after menopause. It is now known that there are different types of estrogen. Women only run out of one type of estrogen at menopause, the type that causes a proliferation of cells in the ovary, womb, and breast in order to bear children. Herbs do not contain the same estrogen as HRT and are usually therefore nonproliferative.

Research into phytoestrogens (plant estrogens) has also shown that phytoestrogens don't simply increase the amount of estrogen in the body, and do not necessarily result in an increase of estrogen at all, but instead bind to receptors on the surface of the cells, and in some scenarios can protect against estrogen excess. In other words, they have a modulation effect.

The estrogen in HRT and the contraceptive pill has the same receptor affinity as our ovarian estrogen; this means that phytoestrogens are not similar to HRT (or the contraceptive pill). Phytoestrogens have an affinity for a different receptor to the estrogen from our ovaries, making them potentially safer and generally nonproliferative.

Herbal remedies are not a natural version of HRT, but can be complementary to HRT and can help treat symptoms that are not responding to HRT. See also Chapter 6.

SEEING AN HERBAL PRACTITIONER

THE CONSULTATION

An herbal practitioner will take a full and detailed case history and look at diet, lifestyle, and health issues that may be impacting menopausal change. Menopause should be about a successful adaptation to lowered estrogen levels, as the ovaries stop playing a major role in hormone regulation. Problems can happen for a mosaic of reasons, especially in relation to digestive health and changes to the nervous system.

AN OVERALL VIEW

To find a practitioner, check with the American Herbalist Guild. Herbalists can give advice about holistic living, diet, and nutrition, but cannot prescribe or treat for any specific condition. You may need to also enlist a physician, a dietitian, and a coach or other provider. It may be possible to focus on changing diet and lifestyle for the better, while using medicinal herbs to benefit the areas of the body that are overstressed.

" "

Approximately 51% of women use complementary and alternative medicine during menopause, and more than 60% perceive it to be effective for menopausal symptoms.

HOLISTIC USE OF HERBAL REMEDIES

Herbal remedies can be applied to the areas of your body that contribute to hormone balance without directly providing estrogen. You can therefore induce benefits by addressing hormone levels or by addressing nervous system health, or both. Herbs such as oat straw (see page 54) or maca root (see page 65) can act over time like tonics to both these systems. An herbal medicine such as lemon balm (see page 45) can reduce stress levels during the day, and when combined with a relaxing herb such as valerian (see page 53) at night, can reduce night sweats without directly influencing estrogen. Better sleep might then increase energy levels and reduce brain fog.

Herbs that help sleep such as lavender (see page 47) or chamomile (see page 49) also have positive benefits for your digestive system, which has a key role to play in menopausal hormone production. Drinking a nutritious, anti-inflammatory herbal tea of dandelion, St. John's wort, and licorice may improve your digestive health so much that you absorb minerals more effectively from your gut, and combined with an improved diet, this can contribute positively to bone density and cardiovascular health. You can also reduce brain fog and boost energy with herbal teas, rather than caffeine, which aggravates hot flashes.

Menopause is the perfect time to look at how you eat, drink, live, work, rest, and relax. It can be revelatory to be guided by a practitioner who will have a unique functional view of the human body and its interconnectedness. This is an opportunity to take back ownership of your own health, and to make changes to address the root causes of menopausal symptoms.

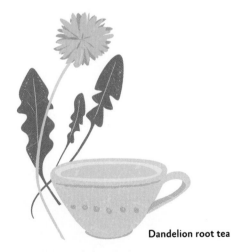

Dandelion root tea

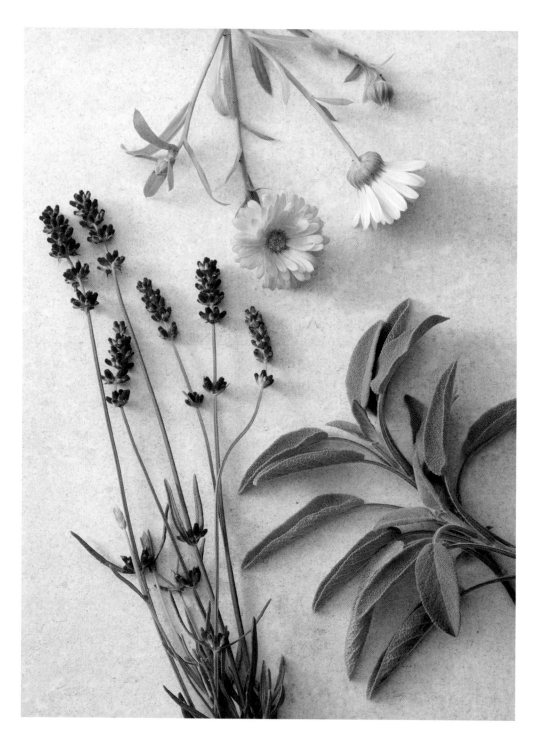

AROMATHERAPY

In aromatherapy there are over 150 different essential oils. Each oil can have up to 100 different chemical components, giving each oil its own unique chemistry, distinct fragrance, and therapeutic properties, both physiological and psychological. The holistic effects of essential oils can help with many menopausal symptoms including anxiety, depression, mood swings, sleep disturbances, headaches, hot flashes, and loss of libido.

Your sense of smell, often underused, is very powerful. When you smell something, your body's response is processed in the limbic part of the brain, where emotions and memories are processed. This is why certain smells can evoke emotional and/or physical responses. In addition, when a woman is experiencing fluctuation in her estrogen levels, this affects the limbic brain, which is why many women experience psychological symptoms during menopause.

Bathing is a great way to get creative with essential oils. Make your morning shower a vitality boost, or turn your bath soak into a spa experience by adding calming geranium essential oil (see page 71).

MASSAGE

Therapeutic massage, especially when using essential oils, has many benefits during menopause. It stimulates blood circulation, so it can help lower blood pressure, activates the body's lymphatic system, reduces fluid retention and swelling, and can reduce pain. Studies show that it helps increase the release of oxytocin, the love hormone, so it can be useful for improving libido and feelings of emotion.

Massage also calms the nervous system, and can help reduce stress, pave the way for better sleep, and ease numerous menopausal symptoms. A face and head massage works wonders for insomnia and headaches, while massaging the abdomen with a sweet fennel massage oil can help relieve bloating (see page 72).

HOW TO USE THIS CHAPTER

This chapter provides useful information about the benefits of key herbal remedies and aromatherapy for menopause, so you can be informed before seeing an herbal practitioner or making your own essential oil blends.

" "

Seek professional advice so that you choose the right herbs or oils for you at menopause. Each herb has its own benefits—for example, sage is known to boost mental clarity, lavender can improve sleep, and marigold soothes skin.

HERBAL REMEDIES

Humans have used herbs as medicine for hundreds of thousands of years. Most women will benefit physically and emotionally from a mixture of herbs that help hormone production and balance, support the digestive and nervous systems, and address imbalances in areas such as the immune system during menopause and beyond.

BENEFITS OF HERBAL REMEDIES

This chapter outlines the main herbs that are shown to be effective for menopause. It looks at the benefits of each herb, which herbs work well together, and how to take them. Some very useful herbal remedies for menopause can be enjoyed as an herb tea or tisane, taken as tinctures or capsules, or applied as a cream.

CONSULTING A KNOWLEDGEABLE PROVIDER

As every woman is different, which herbs to take, and for how long, will vary from person to person, so you should always get advice from a medical provider who will help discover the root cause of your symptoms and provide an individualized treatment.

Addressing hormonal imbalances early is likely to make menopause easier, so a good time to start taking herbal remedies is at perimenopause—or even before—to correct menstrual problems.

Find a provider to guide you who is educated in herbal remedies. When starting an herbal regimen it is important to check with your medical provider, especially if you are taking regular medications.

CAUTIONS

Most herbal remedies are very safe and can be taken for months. However, make sure the herbal product is authentic and from a reputable source. You can also check with your physician for interactions, as well as with your pharmacist.

LEMON BALM

BOOSTS MOOD I IMPROVES SLEEP I CALMS I BENEFITS DIGESTION

Lemon balm (*Melissa officinalis*) has relaxing, anti-inflammatory, and antiviral effects that have made it prominent as a medicine. A member of the mint family, it has an uplifting scent and is ideal for the digestive and nervous systems, which can be negatively affected by menopausal hormone changes.

Lemon balm has been shown to have a positive impact on reducing anxiety and lifting mood, making it ideal for the ups and downs of perimenopause and beyond.

It is gentle on the digestive system, too, and has antispasmodic effects, so it can be useful when there is bloating or digestive upset, which are common symptoms during menopause.

Safe to use regularly, lemon balm is cooling and calming and so for some women it can ease hot flashes and night sweats. It is gently sedative, making it ideal to reduce anxiety and heat during the day, or to aid sleep and minimize night sweats.

HOW IT WORKS

This bright but calming herb restores function of the nervous system and eases the effects of stress on the digestive system.

HOW TO TAKE IT

- **Lemon balm leaves** (either fresh or dried) make a pleasant tea that can be enjoyed in the day to calm, relax, and boost mood, and in the evening to help with sleep.
- **If you prefer,** you can take lemon balm in capsule form.

COMBINES WELL WITH

Lemon balm works via the gut–brain axis to reduce menopausal symptoms, so it is best taken with hormone-balancing herbs such as chaste tree (see page 60) or sage (see page 62), and digestive herbs such as chamomile (see page 49) or lavender (see page 47).

CAUTIONS

If you have low thyroid function, do not use unless you have consulted a physician.

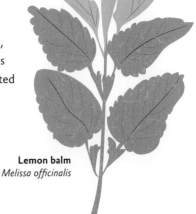

Lemon balm
Melissa officinalis

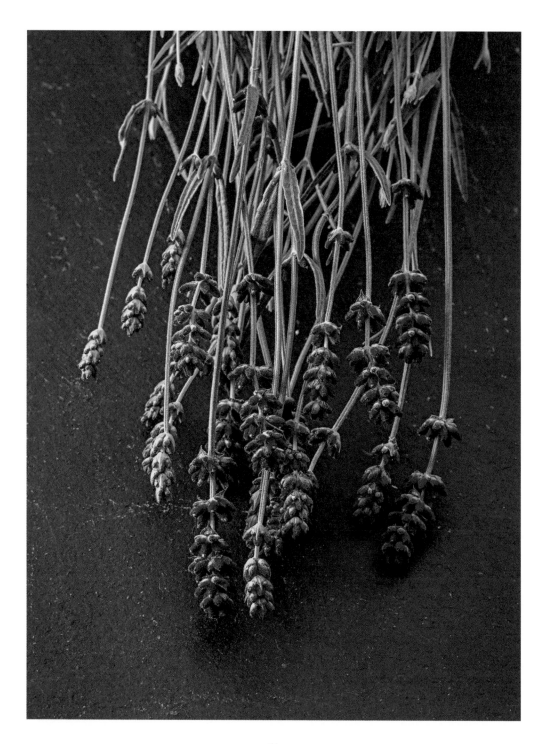

LAVENDER

BENEFITS DIGESTION I SOOTHES HEADACHES I BOOSTS MOOD I SOOTHES SKIN

Lavender (*Lavandula officinalis*) is well known for its aromatic essential oil. The whole herb, however, is used as an aromatic tonic for the digestive system, helping relieve digestive issues that often flare up at menopause. Lavender also helps lift mood and reduce anxiety, and can help with breast tenderness.

Lavender tea or tincture eases discomfort in the digestive system and the head, and is both relaxing and uplifting, so is ideal during menopausal mood changes. It can provide stability when menopausal symptoms are fluctuating, helping with brain fog, mild headaches, and improving mental clarity. Lavender also has positive digestive effects when used as an herbal medicine, soothing bloating, fullness, indigestion, and symptoms of Irritable Bowel Syndrome (IBS), which can worsen or start during menopause.

HOW IT WORKS

In addition to its essential oils, lavender contains mild bitters, antioxidants, and anti-inflammatory compounds.

HOW TO TAKE IT

- **Enjoy a fragrant infusion** of the leaves or flowers in small amounts throughout the day (see box, right).
- **The leaves and flowers** also work well as a compress for inflamed skin or for breast tenderness. Apply externally to red or inflamed skin eruptions, especially around the chin area where acne-type spots can occur during menopause.
- **Lavender can also** be used as a tincture.

COMBINES WELL WITH

Lavender can enhance the effects of hormone-balancing herbs such as chaste tree (see page 60) and black cohosh (see page 61).

CAUTIONS

There are no known cautions.

LAVENDER INFUSION

- A lavender infusion can relieve fullness and ease a mild headache.
- Use ¹⁄₁₀oz (2–4g) of lavender flowers or leaves in 10fl oz (300ml) of water to make a pleasant-tasting infusion.
- Drink twice a day, ideally after a meal, to ease bloating; or when a headache starts.

ST. JOHN'S WORT

BOOSTS AND BALANCES MOOD I REDUCES HOT FLASHES I CALMS

St. John's wort (*Hypericum perforatum*) is traditionally considered a valuable
tonic for the nervous system and combines well with many other herbal
relaxants and uplifting medicinal plants. It can reduce the severity and frequency
of hot flashes and night sweats, and reduce irritability and mood swings.

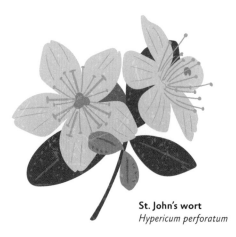

St. John's wort
Hypericum perforatum

HOW IT WORKS

St. John's wort has been investigated for
its antidepressant effects via numerous
pathways. Research shows it can also help
repair the cells of the nervous system.

HOW TO TAKE IT

- **Use the plant** either fresh or dried.
- **Make a tea** from the leaves and flowers.
- **Use capsules** and tablets made from the
whole powdered plant, not isolated extracts.

St. John's wort is valued for its beneficial
effects on the immune system, and for
increasing resilience to recurrent viral
infections. It is also widely used for
emotional upsets and can be very useful
for helping with mood fluctuations, tension,
and anxiety during menopause, as well
as reducing the severity of hot flashes.
One study showed that women had
improved PMS symptoms when using a
combination of St. John's wort and chaste
tree (see page 60).

COMBINES WELL WITH

St. John's wort works well when taken
alongside anxiety-reducing herbs such as
lavender (see page 47), chamomile (see
page 49), and lemon balm (see page 45).

CAUTIONS

Consult a physician, especially before taking
with antidepressant medications as there can
be significant interactions. Avoid long
exposure to sunlight if taking a high dose.
Not suitable for treating serious depression.

CHAMOMILE

IMPROVES SLEEP I BOOSTS MOOD I BENEFITS DIGESTION I SOOTHES SKIN

Chamomile (*Matricaria recutita*) is best known in tea form as aiding restful sleep. It is also anti-inflammatory to the skin and digestive system and is often suggested to treat digestive issues that appear or get worse at menopause as it soothes sore or inflamed membranes in the gut.

Because of the central role of the gut and the nervous system in hormone balance, especially at menopause, chamomile is a key herb. Long-term use can help restore the nervous system to the gut when long-term stress has had a detrimental impact.

Herbalists often combine chamomile with aromatic herbs to help symptoms of bloating or nausea at menopause. Chamomile can be used over a long period of time to help ease anxiety, restlessness, irritability, sleep disruption, and low mood. It has also been shown to be effective for treating skin rashes and vaginal dryness.

HOW IT WORKS

Chamomile contains aromatic essential oils that have anti-inflammatory and antispasmodic effects, plus flavonoids that have wound-healing properties. It also contains specialized mucilages that soothe the digestive membranes and support a healthy gut flora (microbiome).

HOW TO TAKE IT

- **Chamomile can** be taken on its own or combined with other herbs to make a calming tea. It is best taken before bed and is most effective when used regularly.
- **Use as a bathing** herb to ease sore skin.

COMBINES WELL WITH

Chamomile works particularly well with other relaxing herbs such as lavender (see page 47) and lemon balm (see page 45).

CAUTIONS

Seek advice from a physician if you are sensitive to plants in the daisy (*Asteraceae*) family.

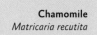

Chamomile
Matricaria recutita

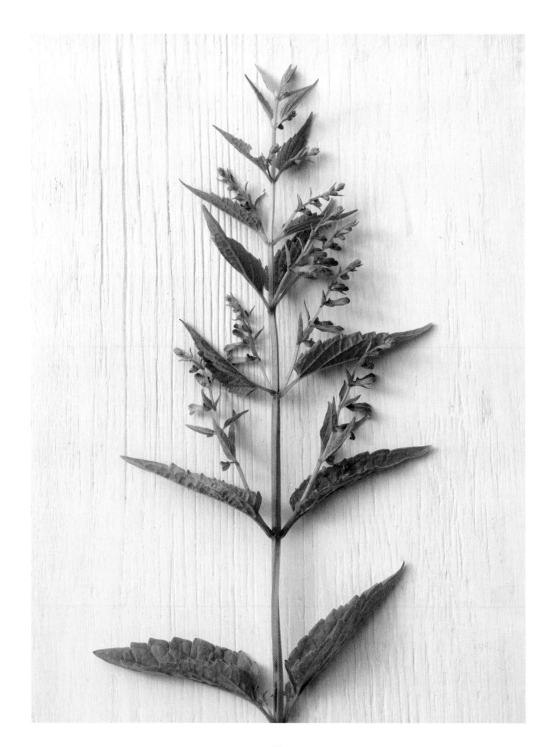

SKULLCAP

BOOSTS AND BALANCES MOOD I IMPROVES SLEEP I REDUCES PALPITATIONS

Skullcap (*Scutellaria lateriflora*) is a gentle nervous system herb with cooling and calming effects on the mind. A member of the mint family, it is well tolerated for extended periods of use. At menopause it can be useful for a busy mind and palpitations that can occur with or without hot flashes.

Skullcap is ideal if you are suffering from restless sleep or if you are feeling hot and irritable, which are common symptoms of menopause. Quieting the emotions and thoughts, this relaxing herb can be ideal if you are feeling overstimulated or overwhelmed with the many changes associated with menopause.

Skullcap has slow, gentle tonic effects on the nervous system, and is best when used regularly over time.

Another species of skullcap (*Scutellaria baicalensis*) has been investigated for its protective properties against breast cancer.

HOW IT WORKS

Like many other members of the mint family, skullcap is thought to work via the sensory nervous system, relaxing you both physically and mentally. This means that although it does not have direct effects on hormone levels, it works indirectly to generally relax the nervous system, reducing palpitations, inflammation, and night sweats.

HOW TO TAKE IT

- **Take every day,** particularly in the morning and evening, for best results. Repeating the dose during the day reminds the body to breathe and calm down, minimizing fluttering thoughts and palpitations.
- **Twice a day** drink an herbal infusion of the leaves and flowers, or take up to ⅙fl oz (5ml) of a simple tincture.
- **Make your own** cooling tea blend: combine skullcap with oat straw (see page 54), lemon balm (see page 45), and lavender flowers (see page 47) in equal parts. Use a teaspoon of the mix in a cup of hot water.

COMBINES WELL WITH

Skullcap is usually combined with soothing herbs such as lemon balm (see page 45) and St. John's wort (see page 48) as the nervous system is more likely to relax when it receives help from multiple sources.

CAUTIONS

It is generally safe for use over long periods.

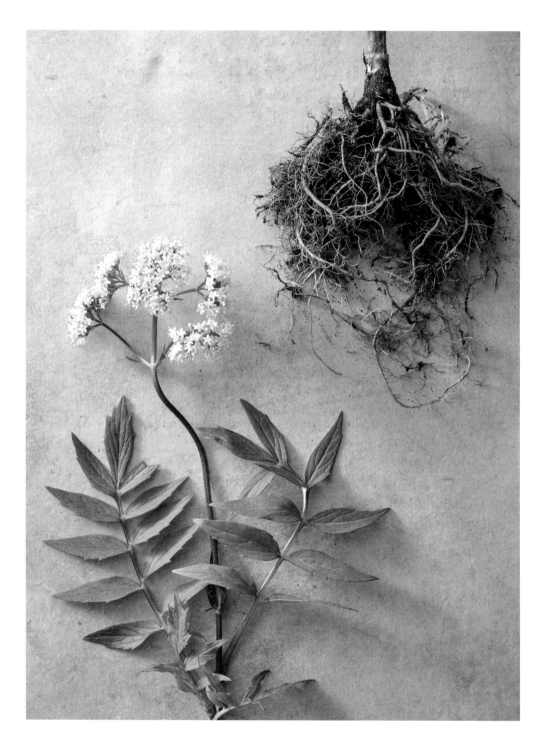

VALERIAN

IMPROVES SLEEP I CALMS I REDUCES HOT FLASHES I BENEFITS DIGESTION

Valerian root (*Valeriana officinalis*) has a long history of use as a sleep aid, and for relief of nervous tension without causing drowsiness or dependency. At menopause it can help restore a connection to good sleep, negate anxious thoughts, and reduce the frequency and intensity of hot flashes.

Used regularly each evening, valerian can help with relaxation and the ability to fall asleep more easily. Several studies show improvements in commonly experienced menopausal symptoms such as anxiety, hot flashes, and night sweats.

Studies show valerian does not have overly sedative effects, so it can be used during the day to ease anxiety or Irritable Bowel Syndrome (IBS) symptoms, as it has antispasmodic effects on the colon.

Valerian's gentle but persistent effects can also have lasting benefits to the nervous system, which is interconnected with female hormones at both menopause and perimenopause.

HOW IT WORKS

Compounds in valerian roots work via neurotransmitters to relax the muscles and reduce restlessness. Relaxant effects on muscular tissues have led to research into its role in easing period pain and other types of muscular pain.

HOW TO TAKE IT

- **Valerian root** has a strong flavor and smell, so it may be easier to take as a tablet or capsule of the powdered root.
- **It can also be taken** in tincture form, or the powdered root can be blended with other relaxing herbs in a tea.
- **Take every night** up to an hour before bed. Effects are usually not instant and may require daily use over several weeks before you see the benefits.

COMBINES WELL WITH

Valerian can reduce hot flashes better when supported by relaxing herbs for the gut and nervous system, such as lavender (see page 47), lemon balm (see page 45), and chamomile (see page 49).

CAUTIONS

Speak with a doctor before combining with antidepressant or anxiety medications. A small number of people report a mildly stimulating rather than relaxing effect.

OAT STRAW

EASES ANXIETY I IMPROVES SLEEP I CALMS I PROVIDES ENERGY

Oat straw (*Avena sativa*), also commonly known as oat flowers or green milky oats, can soothe emotions and strengthen the nervous system. When used regularly it is particularly beneficial for increasing emotional strength as it gradually works over time to increase resilience.

Oat straw is ideal when combined with other nervous system herbs to restore sleep, to increase rejuvenation, and to improve energy levels. It can help reduce the effects of anxiety and stress experienced at menopause when combined with other herbal relaxants, and is not overstimulating, giving a calm inner strength to women who feel worn down by stress or insomnia.

Menopause can be a period of great change, so good sleep and energy levels are very important. Used regularly, over a long period of time, oat straw is an ideal tonic, especially where there are also metabolic problems such as blood sugar imbalances.

Oat straw
Avena sativa

HOW IT WORKS

Oat straw contains a number of important minerals and lipids that help balance blood fat, blood sugar, and hormone levels, as well as supporting the stress response. Oat straw also contains phytoconstituents and glucans that are anti-inflammatory to the skin and nervous system.

HOW TO TAKE IT

- **Use to make** a soft, pleasant-tasting tea.
- **Combine oat straw** with other nervous system tonic herbs, or take regularly morning and evening as a tincture.

COMBINES WELL WITH

Oat straw is a gentle herb that enhances the action of other nervous system tonics such as St. John's wort (see page 48), rosemary (see page 55), and lemon balm (see page 45).

CAUTIONS

Oat straw is generally safe to take over long periods of time.

ROSEMARY

AIDS MEMORY I IMPROVES COGNITION I BOOSTS MOOD I BENEFITS DIGESTION

Rosemary (*Rosmarinus officinalis*) is a familiar culinary herb that has long been associated with preserving memory. Research has suggested it may help with mental clarity and cognitive function, and act as an anti-inflammatory on many tissues of the body, helping manage the aging process and menopause.

Brain fog and poor cognitive function are some of the most commonly reported symptoms of menopause. Rosemary has a long medicinal history for helping improve memory recall, cognition, and mental clarity, as well as possibly reducing the effects of premature aging.

Rosemary is mildly stimulating and tonic, improving circulation to the brain and tissues such as the skin and digestive system. It also has mild immunomodulatory effects and has been investigated for helping prevent recurrent urinary tract infections, which can become more common at menopause.

HOW IT WORKS

Rosemary contains essential oils and compounds that have a mild stimulating and uplifting effect. These are thought to act on the emotional centers of the brain and the endothelium—the lining of the blood vessels where inflammation can originate.

HOW TO TAKE IT

- **Use ¹⁄₁₀oz (1–3g)** of the fresh or dried herb to make an infusion, perfect for a reviving herbal tea. Drink around meal times to optimize digestion and absorption.
- **The pleasant taste** of rosemary means it can be added to food or taken as a tincture.

Rosemary
Rosmarinus Officianalis

COMBINES WELL WITH

Rosemary is often combined with other herbs to improve their absorption; for example, use with dandelion root (see page 67) to aid digestion or with oat straw (see page 54) to improve memory.

CAUTIONS

Use in small therapeutic amounts and do not use for extended periods without having a break.

LICORICE

BOOSTS ENERGY I BALANCES HORMONES I SOOTHES ACHING JOINTS

Licorice root (*Glycyrrhiza glabra*) has a long history of use as a traditional herbal medicine. Although its name means "sweet root," it contains important bitters and other compounds that contribute to its many medicinal effects. It can be used at all stages of menopause to optimize hormone production.

Research confirms that licorice is anti-inflammatory and tissue healing, and supports hormone production, as well as repair of the organs that produce hormones. It can help especially where there is atrophy of tissues such as with vaginal dryness.

Licorice can help at menopause where there is repeated infection, or chronic inflammation, which is impacting menopausal symptoms. It may be useful where there is depletion or lack of energy, and it can help with gastric inflammation.

HOW IT WORKS

Licorice works via numerous mechanisms to achieve broad-spectrum anti-inflammatory and tonic effects. It supports the function of the adrenal glands and therefore the hormones produced there, boosting energy.

HOW TO TAKE IT

- **Licorice is best taken** as a tea (see box, right) or tincture. It has a strong flavor and is often blended with other herbs.

COMBINES WELL WITH

Licorice root is usually combined with other herbs and works best when all areas of the body involved in hormone production are supported. Use with chaste tree (see page 60), black cohosh (see page 61), or red clover (see page 64) to aid menopausal hormones.

CAUTIONS

You can take licorice for short periods, but longer-term use should be monitored by a physician. Large doses or long-term use can cause raised blood pressure, kidney damage, or electrolyte disruptions.

LICORICE AND MINT TEA

- If you are flagging mid-afternoon, try this invigorating infusion.
- Mix ¼–⅓oz (7–10g) of fresh mint with ⅙oz (5g) of powdered licorice root in a teapot. Add 2 cups of hot water. Leave for 5 minutes, strain, and drink.

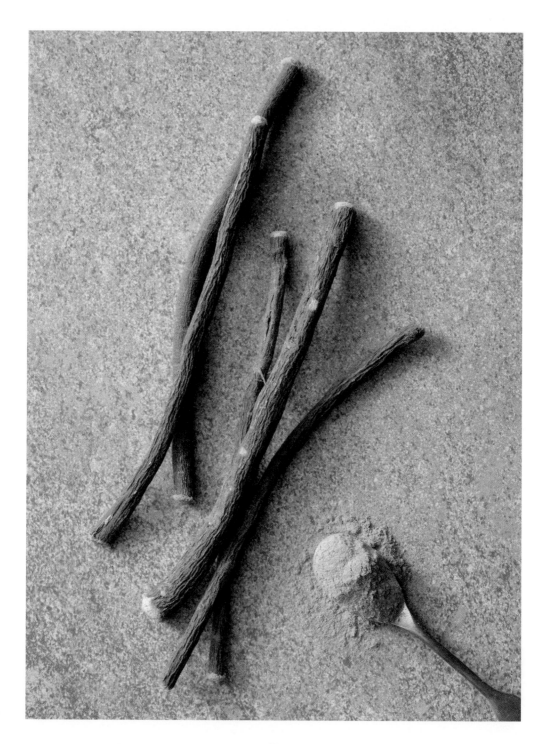

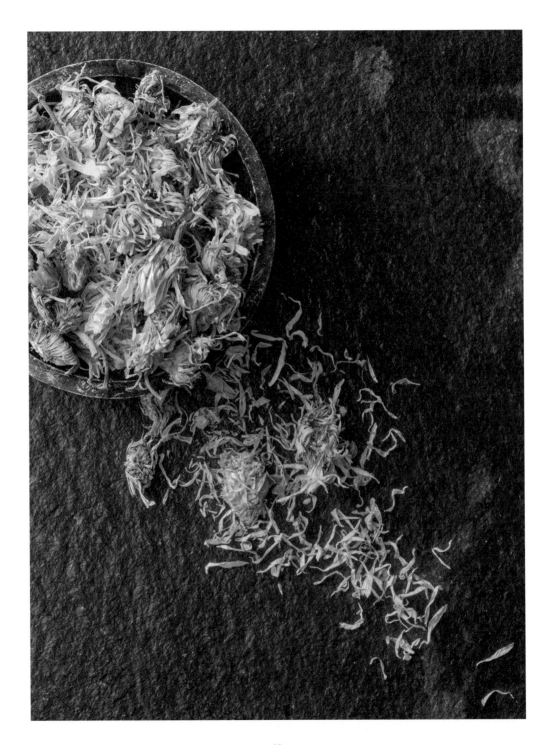

MARIGOLD

SOOTHES SKIN I EASES MENOPAUSAL ACNE I HELPS WOUND HEALING

Marigold (*Calendula officinalis L*), also commonly known as calendula, is a very gentle herbal remedy and is ideal to use at menopause and beyond to relieve infections or swelling. Marigold flowers have been used for centuries as a wound-healing agent, whether applied to the skin or taken internally.

Used in traditional and modern herbalism, marigold can help with many menopausal skin conditions. Today it is commonly used by herbalists for facial acne, recurrent skin infections, and chronic skin congestion such as sebaceous cysts, which can occur at perimenopause. It is also recommended for wound healing, lymphedema after mastectomy, vaginal and vulval atrophy, and vaginal dryness.

HOW IT WORKS

Marigold contains numerous compounds that have a beneficial impact on many different processes at menopause, including lymphatic drainage and wound repair, making it easier for your body's cells to function properly.

HOW TO TAKE IT

■ **Herbal experts use an extraction** of the marigold flowers to make an antifungal and antibacterial cream or pessaries to treat thrush, vaginosis, or vaginal dryness.

■ **Drink an herbal infusion** made from the flower heads or petals once or twice a day.

COMBINES WELL WITH

Marigold's tonic effects on tissues and skin are enhanced when used with other skin tonics such as red clover (see page 64) and licorice (see page 56).

CAUTIONS

Calendula is a very mild and safe remedy unless you have a very rare contact allergy to plants of the daisy (*Asteraceae*) family.

MARIGOLD INFUSION

■ Soothe menopausal skin problems with marigold infusions and infused oils.

■ Make a tea from marigold flowers, leave to cool, then use regularly to bathe acne and tender or sore skin.

■ Use an infused oil of marigold on troublesome spots or dry itchy patches.

CHASTE TREE

BOOSTS AND BALANCES MOOD I REGULATES HORMONES I ALLEVIATES PMS

Chaste tree (*Vitex agnus castus*) has been used for centuries to treat premenstrual symptoms. It is now recognized as an effective herbal remedy for managing a wide range of menopausal complaints because it helps balance hormone levels and normalize the ratio of progesterone to estrogen.

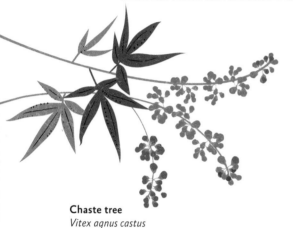

Chaste tree
Vitex agnus castus

Chaste tree is most commonly used for menstrual disorders, and most research has been into how it can reduce the symptoms of PMS. It has been proven that taking chaste tree has helped some women with a number of menopausal symptoms, including headaches, fatigue, and mood swings.

HOW IT WORKS

Chaste tree is classed as an amphoteric, which means that it balances out hormonal changes. Although it does not contain

hormones, it works via the pituitary gland at the base of the brain, balancing secretions of hormones from there, which in turn helps rebalance estrogen and progesterone levels. As hormone levels fluctuate during menopause, this can help maintain overall balance and mood.

HOW TO TAKE IT

- **Chaste tree berries** are commonly dried to a powder and taken orally in tablet form.
- **If buying a powdered extract,** ensure it contains the berry/fruit part of the plant.
- **Chaste tree is also available** as a tincture.

COMBINES WELL WITH

Chaste tree works well with herbs such as chamomile (see page 49), which supports the liver as it processes hormones.

CAUTIONS

Side effects are extremely rare at normal dosage, but high doses have been found to cause transient headaches.

BLACK COHOSH

REDUCES HOT FLASHES I BOOSTS AND BALANCES MOOD I IMPROVES SLEEP

Black cohosh (*Actaea racemosa*) is used therapeutically to help alleviate a number of common symptoms of menopause. Traditionally used by Native American herbalists, it can be particularly effective at minimizing the more severe effects of hot flashes and night sweats.

Research has found that black cohosh can alleviate painful menstrual cramps and help with debilitating mood changes.

HOW IT WORKS
Studies show black cohosh works via a variety of mechanisms to alleviate menopausal symptoms, and illustrates the interconnectedness of different parts of the body in maintaining hormone balance. It does not interact with estrogen receptors as was previously thought. It works partly by modifying pituitary hormones and neurotransmitter activity, thus having benefits to the brain and nervous system that could account for improvements in mood, anxiety, and insomnia.

HOW TO TAKE IT
■ **Buy tablets, tinctures, or herbal teas** made from the dried root and rhizomes of the black cohosh plant.
■ **It is advisable to take** black cohosh with food to reduce the risk of stomach upsets.

■ **It is essential that** you buy a registered product so that it is pure and has not been contaminated by other plants.

COMBINES WELL WITH
As black cohosh aids the nervous system, it works well with herbs that are restorative to the nervous system such as valerian (see page 53), chamomile (see page 49), and St. John's wort (see page 48).

CAUTIONS
Black cohosh has a good safety record at normal dose. Excessive doses may cause digestive disturbance, dizziness, or headaches. Avoid if you have a liver condition, unless monitored by a medical practitioner.

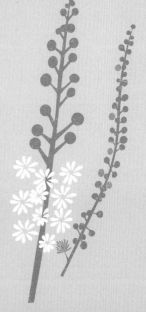

Black cohosh
Actaea racemosa

SAGE

SUPPORTS METABOLISM | REDUCES HOT FLASHES | IMPROVES COGNITION

Sage (*Salvia officinalis*) is a well-known culinary herb. "Salvia" means "healing," and sage's antioxidant and anti-inflammatory properties are effective for treating many common menopausal symptoms. Sage (meaning "wise") also has positive effects on brain function and may improve memory recall.

A recent study found that taking sage every day reduced the severity of hot flashes, with half the women in the study finding their hot flashes had decreased after taking sage for four weeks.

Sage has traditionally been used as a remedy for sore throats and gums. As some women become more susceptible to recurrent infections at perimenopause or begin to experience sensitive teeth and gum disease after menopause, sage can be a useful tonic.

Studies have also shown that sage can have beneficial effects on cholesterol and blood-sugar levels.

HOW IT WORKS

Sage contains antioxidants, antimicrobials, and anti-inflammatories that may help reduce excessive stress on the body, reducing sweating and decreasing hot flashes. It is not yet clear how it helps reduce hot flashes because it does not contain estrogen.

HOW TO TAKE IT

- **Sage leaves** can be made into an herbal infusion (see box, below).
- **Sage** can also be taken in a tincture.

COMBINES WELL WITH

Sage is more effective for hot flashes when the nervous system is also supported with herbs such as St. John's wort (see page 48).

CAUTIONS

As sage contains thujone, having too much or for too long may cause rashes or vomiting. Do not take if pregnant or you have epilepsy.

SAGE TEA

- Pour 1 cup of boiling water over 1 tablespoon of fresh sage leaves and cover to capture the aromas.
- Leave to steep for 4–5 minutes, then strain out the leaves.
- Enjoy while hot, or add fruit juice, chill, and drink throughout the day.

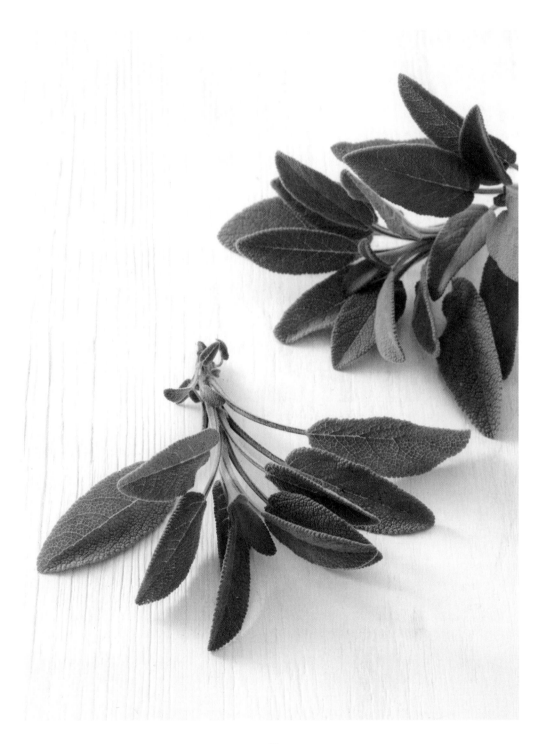

RED CLOVER

REDUCES HOT FLASHES I BOOSTS TISSUE ELASTICITY I SOOTHES SKIN

Red clover (*Trifolium pratense*) is an effective herbal remedy for symptoms such as hot flashes. Traditionally it has been used as a nourishing skin tonic to treat eczema and dermatitis, and it can also help maintain healthy hair, skin, and nails, which can all be affected during menopause.

Like soy, red clover is a member of the bean family and contains useful isoflavones, plant-derived compounds similar to those found in soy. As a result, red clover has been investigated for its potential role in helping maintain bone density, and for its benefits on postmenopausal cardiovascular health. It is used for lymphatic drainage and is especially healing to breast tissue. Red clover may provide relief for vaginal atrophy and help with vaginal dryness or recurrent vaginal infections.

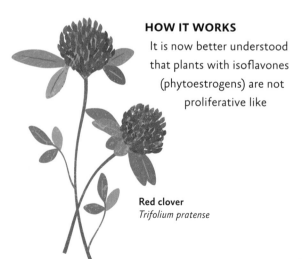

HOW IT WORKS

It is now better understood that plants with isoflavones (phytoestrogens) are not proliferative like estrogen, and may instead act to block estrogen in certain circumstances. Research has shown that phytoestrogens can ease hot flashes and help with libido, low mood, and tiredness, while having potential improvements for bone density, cholesterol, blood pressure, and blood sugar levels. See also page 149.

HOW TO TAKE IT

■ **Take tablets or capsules** of standardized extracts of red clover.

■ **It may prove** more beneficial to use the whole plant and take as a tea or tincture.

COMBINES WELL WITH

Red clover's effects are enhanced when used with tissue tonic herbs such as maca root (see page 65) and marigold (see page 59).

CAUTIONS

Consult a physician before using if you have had a hormone-responsive disease, including breast cancer or endometrial cancer.

Red clover
Trifolium pratense

MACA ROOT

IMPROVES LIBIDO I PROVIDES ENERGY I AIDS CONCENTRATION

Native to the Peruvian Andes, maca root (*Lepidium meyenii/Lepidium peruvianum*) has tonic and nourishing qualities. Sometimes called Peruvian ginseng, it is well known across Latin America for boosting energy levels, libido, and sexual function in both women and men.

Maca root has gentle stimulating and nourishing qualities that have been traditionally used to help improve fertility and sex drive. It can have a gradual but sustained effect on improving the health and vitality of tissues of the body—the skin, muscles, and sex organs.

Maca can act as a tonic for women during menopause, helping with low libido, tiredness, and poor concentration. As it aids convalescence, it is ideal for those who are recovering from a long or chronic illness, or who have low energy or weakness during menopause.

HOW IT WORKS

As with other herbs containing plant sterols, maca root can balance out hormone levels by reducing hormones that are in excess and boosting hormones that are depleted. The body can take what it needs and use the compounds in the plant to help with normal processes of hormone production and breakdown.

HOW TO TAKE IT

- **Have a small teaspoon** of the powdered root daily. It's delicious, and can easily be added to everyday foods such as muesli, yogurt, or smoothies.
- **Take maca root** in the daytime for energy, then take herbal relaxants (see below) at night to reinforce a good day–night rhythm.

Maca root
*Lipidium meyenii/
Lipidium peruvianum*

COMBINES WELL WITH

Maca root restores nervous system balance when combined with relaxants such as valerian (see page 53), lavender (see page 47), or lemon balm (see page 45).

CAUTIONS

Can have an impact on thyroid function.

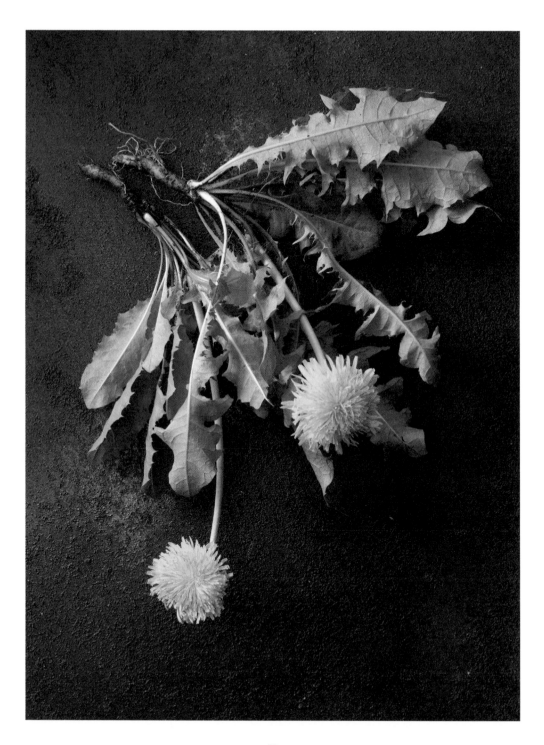

DANDELION

BENEFITS DIGESTION I ALLEVIATES CONSTIPATION I PROVIDES ENERGY

Dandelion (*Taraxacum officinale*) is an important medicinal herb around the globe, and is really three medicines in one plant (leaf, root, and flower). It can be applied to almost any ailment, but at menopause it is the root that can be particularly helpful in ensuring better hormone balance via digestive health.

Dandelion root can be helpful if you are prone to erratic or sluggish bowel habits or feel bloated and full around the middle, and it can be beneficial if you have been anemic or tired due to low iron reserves, all of which can be issues at menopause.

Dandelion has a number of positive applications, especially when there is an imbalance of hormones. Traditionally used as a skin clearing and tonic herb, it helps clear congestion by improving liver function and elimination of normal waste products of metabolism.

HOW IT WORKS

Dandelion helps the function of the liver, which is involved in post-menopausal hormone homeostasis (the cycle of hormone manufacture and elimination). It improves absorption of—and is rich in—the nutrients that help nourish the blood and prevent mineral loss. Research also shows that it benefits the microbiome—now recognized as important in hormone balance.

HOW TO TAKE IT

- **Dandelion root** can be made into a tea from the powder, or roasted and brewed somewhat like coffee because it has a bittersweet flavor.
- Use $\frac{1}{10}$–$\frac{1}{6}$oz (2–5g) of powdered root once or twice daily to give a gentle nudge to the digestive system and help improve nutrition, liver detoxification, and thus skin health and overall energy.

COMBINES WELL WITH

Dandelion improves mineral absorption and hormone balance when used with aromatic herbs such as rosemary (see page 55) and lavender (see page 47).

CAUTIONS

Dandelion is safe to consume over long periods of time. Excessive doses may temporarily cause looser bowel movements, but this is a foodlike herb and it is safe to use alongside medication. For best results it may be necessary to include the leaf as well as the root.

ESSENTIAL OILS

Aromatherapy is one of the most widely used natural remedies. A regular, soothing massage from a qualified aromatherapist and using essential oils everyday are nurturing and effective ways to ease many perimenopausal and menopausal symptoms. Essential oils can help boost mood and libido, calm stress and anxiety, improve sleep, and reduce hot flashes and brain fog.

BUYING AND STORING OILS

Always buy pure, natural, good-quality essential oils and check the botanical name to ensure you are buying the correct oil. Keep in a dark and cool place to maximize their life and therapeutic properties.

USING AND BLENDING OILS

The quickest way to access the power of aromatherapy is through inhalation—simply inhaling essential oils from a tissue, an aromastick, a rollerball, or a diffuser. You can also massage a blended oil into your skin, which rejuvenates the mind and body; or use aromatic bathing products to keep your skin nourished and hydrated.

Self-massage with essential oils is detoxing, improving skin health and tone by encouraging good circulation and eliminating impurities. It is also beneficial for many menopausal symptoms—a face and head massage can help with insomnia or headaches, while massaging the abdomen can help with digestive issues. You can also use a compress infused with essential oils to soothe and calm specific painful areas.

If blending, choose two or three oils that you like and have the needed properties, like oils for relaxation, energy, or boosting libido.

CAUTIONS

People with asthma should take care when inhaling oils, especially if diffused. Never ingest oils or apply them undiluted to skin, and seek medical advice if oil goes in your eye. Do a patch test before using.

CLARY SAGE

REDUCES HOT FLASHES I BOOSTS MOOD I EASES ANXIETY I IMPROVES LIBIDO

Clary sage (*Salvia sclarea*) essential oil is renowned for its calming, balancing, and uplifting properties. A wonderful essential oil, it is used to treat many aspects of women's health by balancing hormones and helping alleviate hot flashes, night sweats, and loss of libido during menopause.

Clary sage lifts mood and calms irritability, depression, and anxiety. It can help restore feelings of vitality and well-being, and its antispasmodic action helps relieve painful periods. As a hormone balancer, it can help you cope with hot flashes along with loss of libido.

HOW IT WORKS

Clary sage is rich in esters, which are known for their antispasmodic and sedative properties. Plus, it contains estrogenic substances that help balance hormones.

HOW TO USE IT
- **Use diluted** in a bath oil or massage oil.
- **Use in a diffuser** or a spritz (see box).

BLENDS WELL WITH

The scent of clary sage is sweet, herbaceous, and warm. It blends well with bergamot (see page 74), all citrus oils, juniper, jasmine, sandalwood, cedarwood, atlas, and basil.

CAUTIONS

There are no known cautions. It's nontoxic, nonirritant in dilution, and nonsensitizing.

SPRITZ FOR HOT FLASHES

Use this mix of cooling and calming essential oils at the start of a hot flash.

- Put 3fl oz (100ml) of rosewater in a spritz bottle with these essential oils: 3 drops of clary sage; 3 drops of geranium; and 4 drops of bergamot. Spritz on the chest when required.

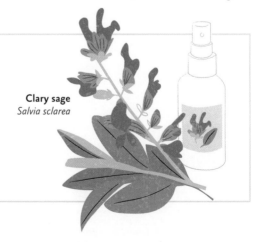

Clary sage
Salvia sclarea

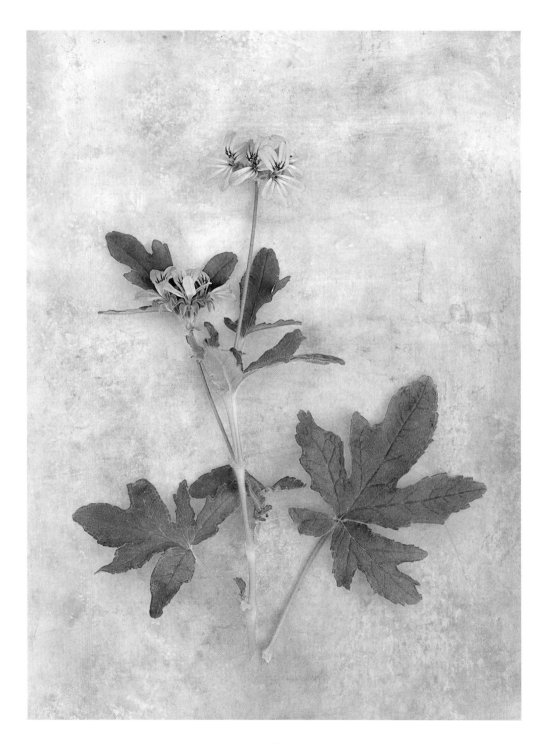

GERANIUM

BOOSTS MOOD I REDUCES HOT FLASHES I SOOTHES SKIN I IMPROVES SLEEP

Geranium *(Pelargonium graveolens)* essential oil is renowned for its balancing and harmonizing properties, helping calm and lift your mood and regulate emotions. This is a helpful essential oil for menopausal skin issues as it has anti-inflammatory properties and can soothe topsy-turvy hormonal skin.

If you are feeling hot-headed, irritable, restless, or anxious, geranium can cool, calm, and center your emotions, promoting a positive outlook. As a hormone balancer it helps with hot flashes, and it also encourages circulation, so it is useful if you suffer from fluid retention or heavy periods during perimenopause.

HOW IT WORKS

This floral oil's chemical properties make its prime therapeutic actions very supportive to menopausal symptoms. Geranium helps the body harmonize and balance, making it an effective detoxifying, skin-regulating, and anti-inflammatory agent. It is a key hormone balancer, assisting with emotional swings, and may also help lower blood pressure.

HOW TO USE IT

- **Place a few drops** on a tissue and inhale when you want to feel calm.
- **Blend with other oils** to make a relaxing bath oil or massage oil (see box).

BLENDS WELL WITH

Geranium is a powerful scent with sweet, rosy, leafy green, slightly minty notes. It blends well with all citrus and floral oils, including mandarin and rose (see page 77), as well as spicy, herby, and woody scented oils.

CAUTIONS

There are no known cautions. It is nontoxic, nonirritant in dilution, and nonsensitizing.

MASSAGE OIL FOR CALM

Use this soothing and balancing massage oil to calm yourself at the end of the day and prepare for a good night's sleep.

- Put 1fl oz (30ml) of grapeseed oil in a small bottle, and then add the following essential oils: 6 drops of geranium, 6 drops of lavender, and 3 drops of Roman chamomile. Put the lid on and combine well.
- Use this fragrant blend for a therapeutic massage in the evening.

SWEET FENNEL

EASES BLOATING I PROVIDES ENERGY I CALMS I BOOSTS MOOD

The essential oil of sweet fennel *(Foeniculum vulgare)* is produced from the distillation of the crushed seeds from its golden yellow flowers. Sweet fennel has a long history as a medicinal herb dating back to the Greeks and Romans, and is particularly helpful to relieve menopausal bloating and feelings of heaviness.

Sweet fennel oil benefits the nervous system and is a tonic oil to lift your spirits and let go of any negative feelings with its fresh, sweet, and refreshing aroma.

HOW IT WORKS

The oil contains mildly estrogenic substances that help balance hormones and can alleviate symptoms such as an irregular menstrual cycle, water retention, irritability, and fatigue. As a strong diuretic it works well on the lymphatic systems if you are prone to swelling and water retention at menopause. It also aids a sluggish digestive system, helping with bloating.

HOW TO USE IT

- **Place a few drops** on a tissue and inhale directly to relax the mind.
- **Add to a diffuser** or a spritz.
- **Use in a massage oil** to ease bloating and abdominal discomfort (see box, left).
- **Use as a chest rub** to help quell feelings of irritability and balance emotions.

BLENDS WELL WITH

Sweet fennel has a distinctive fresh, sweet, peppery aroma with hints of aniseed. It blends well with geranium (see page 71), rose (see page 77), and minty and citrus oils.

CAUTIONS

Avoid if pregnant. Sweet fennel oil is nonirritant in dilution and nonsensitizing.

MASSAGE OIL TO SOOTHE THE ABDOMEN

Use this hormone-balancing massage oil to relieve uncomfortable bloating.

- Put 1fl oz (30ml) of grapeseed oil in a bottle, then add the following essential oils: 5 drops of sweet fennel, 6 drops of geranium (see page 71), and 4 drops of peppermint. Put the lid on and shake.
- Massage slowly and gently onto your abdominal area in a clockwise direction.

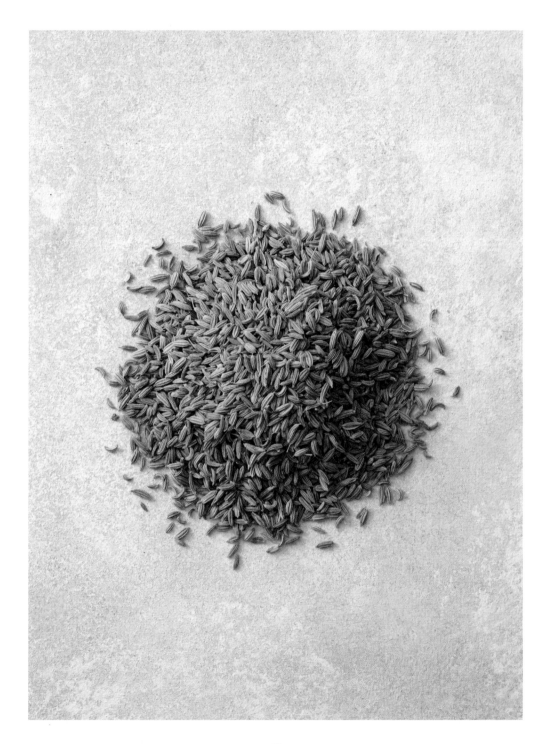

BERGAMOT

BOOSTS MOOD I CALMS I BENEFITS DIGESTION I SOOTHES HEADACHES

Bergamot oil (*Citrus bergamia*) is famously known for giving Earl Grey tea
its distinctive flavor. It is relaxing yet distinctly uplifting, making it a useful
oil to ease many of the psychological symptoms of menopause. In particular,
it encourages the release of feelings of frustration and irritability.

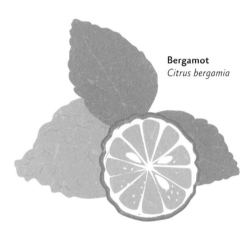

Bergamot
Citrus bergamia

Bergamot oil is a perfect pick-me-up
remedy, evoking feelings of joy and
well-being. It can help you stay calm,
reducing the emotions that often lead to
anxiety, depression, and insomnia. It is also
helpful for headaches, nervous indigestion,
and loss of appetite due to stress.

HOW IT WORKS

Bergamot oil comes from the cold expression
of the rind of the bergamot orange; and like
all citrus oils, it is cooling and refreshing.

HOW TO USE IT

■ **Place 1–2 drops** on a tissue and inhale, or
use in a diffuser to help create feelings of
relaxed alertness.
■ **Bergamot is a versatile oil** and can be
added to massage oil and bath products.
■ **Apply to your pulse points** in a blend
throughout the day to keep you calm,
level-headed, and motivated. It can also
help relieve tension headaches.
■ **Use in a body spritz** to promote a calm
and clear mind.

BLENDS WELL WITH

The scent of bergamot is sweet and fruity
with a fresh green note. It blends well with
most other essential oils, making it a staple
for any aromatherapy box.

CAUTIONS

Use bergapten-free bergamot oil (FCF)
to avoid problems with sunlight exposure.
It is nontoxic, nonirritant in dilution,
and nonsensitizing.

CYPRESS

CALMS I REDUCES HOT FLASHES I EASES BLOATING I SOOTHES SKIN

Cypress oil (*Cupressus sempervirens*) is obtained from the needlelike leaves of the iconic Mediterranean tree. Known as a transition oil, it can help you move forward in times of menopausal change. It can also help strengthen an overburdened nervous system and restore feelings of calm.

This is a key essential oil for circulation, and its astringent effects make it particularly supportive for menopausal symptoms such as heavy periods, hot flashes, night sweats, and excessive perspiration.

Cypress is refreshing and can help ease frayed nerves and weariness.

HOW IT WORKS

Cypress oil has diuretic properties, so it can reduce water retention and bloating. It can balance and calm oily and congested skin, helping menopausal acne, and can help regulate the menstrual cycle. It also has antispasmodic actions to alleviate painful periods during perimenopause.

HOW TO USE IT

- **Cypress oil** is a very versatile oil and can be inhaled or used in both massage and bath oil blends.
- **Blend with lavender** and clary sage (see page 69) in a warm compress to soothe abdominal cramps and ease heavy periods.

- **Use in a diffuser** to reduce hot flushes.
- **Add to a foot bath** to cool hot feet.

BLENDS WELL WITH

This woody oil has a sweet, earthy but fresh scent of a pine forest and the Mediterranean. It blends well with most oils, especially sweet orange, geranium (see page 71), sweet marjoram, lavender, and grapefruit.

CAUTIONS

There are no known cautions. It is nontoxic, nonirritant in dilution, and nonsensitizing.

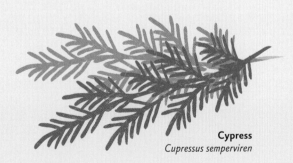

Cypress
Cupressus semperviren

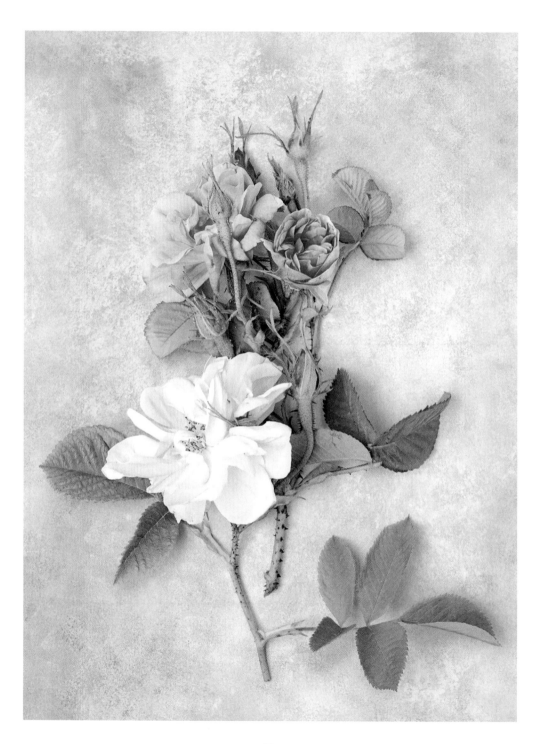

ROSE

BOOSTS MOOD I IMPROVES SLEEP I SOOTHES SKIN I IMPROVES LIBIDO I CALMS

Rose (*Rosa damascena*) is a beautifully floral essential oil that supports femininity and the nervous system. Giving a sweet, gentle comfort, it will help you feel nurtured and build your capacity for self-love during menopause, allowing you the space to experience joy and release sexual energy.

Roses have been used throughout history for their calming and uplifting aroma, and this precious essential oil comes from the distillation of the petals of the rose flower. Its calming properties are helpful for palpitations, irritability, feelings of frustration, and insomnia.

HOW IT WORKS

Rose oil is cool and calming in nature, and is a wonderful oil for inflamed, unbalanced, and sensitive skin, which is a common symptom of menopause. It is a tonic for the uterus, helping ease heavy, painful periods during perimenopause.

HOW TO USE IT

- **This is a wonderful oil** for all applications, and works very well in a massage oil for the body or face (see box, right).
- **Add a few drops** to a tissue to inhale directly when feeling anxious, so you can benefit from its calming properties.
- **Use** in a spritz to cool hot flashes.

BLENDS WELL WITH

Rose oil has a rich, deep, full-bodied aroma, like the scent of a fresh rose in summer. It blends well with many oils, especially woody, citrus, herby, and other floral oils.

CAUTIONS

There are no known cautions. It is nontoxic, nonirritant in dilution, and nonsensitizing.

FACIAL OIL TO NOURISH

Enjoy the calming scent of this blend and feel your skin soothed and nourished.

- Mix together ⅔fl oz (20ml) of apricot kernel oil, and 1 teaspoon each of calendula macerated oil and rosehip oil in a small bottle.
- Add 2 drops each of the following essential oils: rose, lavender, and cypress (see page 75) and combine.
- Massage 2–4 drops on your face morning and evening after cleansing to moisturize and soothe your skin.

MENTAL
WELLNESS

INTRODUCTION

Menopause can be a time of positive transformation. It can be challenging, too, but with the right information, advice, and support it can provide the ideal opportunity for you to reflect and reconnect with long-forgotten dreams and desires, embrace new ideas, and create the roadmap to the life you want to live.

It's important to remember that every woman's menopause will be different, but whatever your experience, having the knowledge and support to be able to take control of any symptoms is key not only to physical health but also to continued mental health and wellness and ultimately to empower you to plan for the next stage of your life.

Menopause can be an ideal opportunity for a midlife pit stop; a chance to reflect and consider how your priorities may have changed. While the life that you have lived so far may have served you well, it's important to allow yourself the luxury of time to enable you to take stock of your position and discover what may serve you even better going forward.

Menopause can offer exciting opportunities for you to explore fresh interests or focus on a new passion or purpose. Embracing this stage is key to ensuring that you make these years some of the happiest, healthiest, and most fulfilling of your life.

MENOPAUSE AND MENTAL HEALTH

Anyone who has experienced premenstrual syndrome will be well aware of the emotional roller-coaster that fluctuating hormones can cause, but many are simply not prepared for the variety and intensity of symptoms that affect some women during menopause. All too often the mental and emotional symptoms of menopause are incorrectly diagnosed as depression and medicated with antidepressants. Being labeled as depressed when you know that you aren't, but don't understand why you feel the way that you do, can be frightening.

Hormones can't take all the blame, though. For the majority of women menopause comes at a time in their lives when many will be juggling the competing responsibilities of family, work, and home life. It can also coincide with the additional responsibility of caring for elderly relatives, older children returning to live at home, and—for some—the ending of long-term relationships. Set this combination against the backdrop of the ever-increasing speed

" "

Every woman's menopause will be different, but having the right
information at the right time can make all the difference in successfully
managing the menopause transition. Every woman deserves to feel
supported and to be able to make the choices that are right for her.

and constant demands and connectivity
of 21st-century life and negative social
attitudes toward menopause and aging, and
it is not surprising that some women feel
overwhelmed when hormone levels begin to
fluctuate during perimenopause.

UNDERSTANDING STRESS

Human beings have a range of physical and
emotional needs, which include autonomy,
security, connection, and purpose among
others. When these are not in balance, this
can lead to both physical and emotional
distress, which can cause both stress and
anxiety. Background stress levels can play an
important part in how we view menopause:
having a clear understanding of why we
experience stress and anxiety in the first
place, and the role that hormones play in
that, can help us understand what is
happening and decide when is the right time
to seek help if we need it.

The brain can be very loosely viewed as
rational or emotional. The rational brain is
in charge of logical thinking and is ideally

in control for the majority of the time. The
emotional brain is in charge of reaction, or
our fight-or-flight response, and the more
stressed you are the more likely that your
emotional brain will take center stage,
often resulting in even more stress.

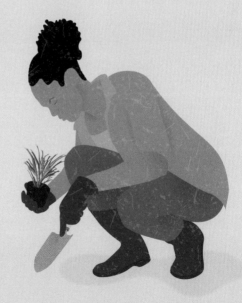

HOW TO MANAGE STRESS AND ANXIETY

BREATHE

Begin and end each day with a simple breathing exercise (see page 91). Focusing on the breath can have a profound effect in helping reduce background stress levels.

PAUSE

When you get up, spend just five minutes in the garden or by an open window and enjoy the stillness of the outdoors. Too often we rush into the day without grounding ourselves first.

TECH DETOX

Switch off the notifications on your phone as they are invasive and trigger the emotional part of the brain. Make the active decision to choose when to respond. See also page 98.

DELEGATE JOBS

Ask yourself if you are doing too much. Have you taken responsibility for things that could be done by other people? Decide what they are and delegate to allow you to take back some time.

ENJOY HOBBIES

When did you last relax and do something that you love, just for you? Reconnect with long-forgotten interests such as gardening, painting, writing, singing, dancing, baking, crafting, or yoga.

SELF-CARE

Focus on your own health and wellness as a priority. Is now the right time to research professional support to help you navigate the menopause transition, or to consider self-help techniques?

FEELING STRETCHED OR STRESSED?

There is a very big difference between feeling stretched and feeling stressed. Feeling stretched gives us meaning and purpose in our lives, a reason to get up in the morning and the fulfilment of rising to the challenge and achieving, which allows us to thrive. When the daily demands on our time and resources become more than we can comfortably cope with, we start to feel negative, defeated, and anxious. Being stretched quickly turns into being stressed, and when that happens life can rapidly start to feel overwhelming and unbalanced, particularly when combined with the hormonal fluctuations of menopause. Identifying stresses and knowing what you can do about them (see box, above) can help.

UNDERSTANDING ANXIETY

Anxiety is one of a series of commonly reported menopause symptoms, and that's because estrogen has a key part to play in brain function. The brain is full of estrogen receptors that help support a variety of functions including cognitive, intellectual, and emotional.

Fluctuating and finally reducing levels of estrogen in the brain during menopause essentially results in an estrogen deficiency, which can cause symptoms such as anxiety, low mood, feeling depressed, mood swings, crying, irritability, anger, loss of confidence, loss of joy, feeling lost, feeling alone, brain fog, memory problems, and poor concentration.

If women are already feeling stressed or anxious, or both, before menopause comes along, then hormone fluctuations will simply compound that situation. So, stress can cause anxiety but continued anxiety can lead to increasing stress levels. Add in hormone fluctuations and menopause symptoms and life can quickly feel overwhelming. A recent study found 48 percent of women aged 50–55 said that their mental health was negatively affected by their menopause symptoms and 25 percent said it made them want to stay at home. It is therefore vital to understand what might be going on, who can help, and—more importantly—how you can help yourself (see box, opposite).

MENOPAUSE AND RELATIONSHIPS

Communication is vital in all our personal and professional relationships, and this is never more important than during menopause. If a woman does not understand what is happening to her it can be hard to talk about what she is experiencing and feeling. It is also important to remember that it is likely that those around her don't understand any changes in behavior of the person they know and love. Even if they don't understand, do everything that you can to keep the lines of communication open as a lack of communication particularly between partners can lead to feelings of confusion and isolation.

" "

If women who are being affected by menopause don't understand what is happening, how can their partners and those around them? Keeping the lines of communication open is vital to ensuring that relationships can weather the menopause storm and emerge stronger and wiser.

PERSONAL RELATIONSHIPS

In a survey for the British Menopause Society, 51 percent of respondents said that their menopause symptoms had affected their sex lives; 38 percent of partners said that they felt helpless to support their partner going through menopause; and 28 percent said this caused arguments. Many loving couples may drift apart both physically and emotionally simply due to a lack of knowledge about menopause. If talking is just too difficult, write a note for your loved ones explaining how you feel and enclose some factual information about menopause to help them understand a little more. Most important of all, tell them how they can support you and how much their support means to you.

RELATIONSHIPS AT WORK

Trying to navigate menopause in the workplace can be challenging if you are struggling with brain fog, lack of concentration, memory lapses, or reduced self-confidence. In a recent survey, 59 percent of working women between the ages of 45 and 55 said menopause had a negative impact on them at work, 65 percent said they were less able to concentrate, and 58 percent said they experienced more stress. Encouragingly, more and more employers are becoming aware of how to support staff experiencing menopause.

If you are planning to speak to your employer it is useful to come up with ideas of what would help you, whether it is the opportunity to work from home, to have flexible hours, to have access to a quiet space during the day, or to be closer to a window for fresh air and ventilation.

Bear in mind that this might be the first time your manager has had this conversation, so give them time to come up with a plan that works for both parties and come back to you to discuss this. Helping others can also be a very positive way of dealing with menopause symptoms in the workplace.

SEEKING PROFESSIONAL SUPPORT

There is no doubt that menopause can be a significant psychological shift in a woman's life, and women often feel the need to stop

Reaching out for support is not a sign of weakness but a sign of strength—
it shows incredible insight. The desire to make the journey through the
menopause transition with the support of another is simply an indication
of the value that you place on the third stage of your life.

and reflect. Many women wish to work through issues that they have identified as having held them back in the past to allow them to move forward and create the life they truly want. It is important to give yourself permission to take this time.

When you decide to seek support, who you turn to will depend on what you are looking to achieve. If you want help to manage your menopause symptoms, then your doctor, menopause specialist, or complementary practitioner will probably be your first port of call. However, if you are looking for support to help you work through how you are feeling, the choice can seem overwhelming. Whoever you choose, whether it's a counselor, coach, psychotherapist, or psychologist, before you see them make sure that they understand menopause and the power of hormones and have some formal training in the subject.

Your practitioner should be able to explain things to you in clear, easy-to-understand language, arming you with the practical skills, tools, and strategies that will allow you to thrive going forward. The choices you make now will help you explore and define your ideal future; you owe it to yourself to make them good ones.

MENOPAUSE COUNSELING

WHY SEE A COUNSELOR?

Sometimes we all need someone to talk to. Seeing a menopause counselor can offer the opportunity to talk about what you are experiencing in a confidential, safe, nonjudgmental environment. Talking to someone who understands can be a welcome relief and provides space and time for you to explore a midlife spring cleaning. It's a chance to consider what is working in your life to enrich it, what isn't, and the changes that you might make going forward.

HOW COUNSELING HELPS

Having someone to support you and reassure you that you are not alone or losing your mind can bring profound relief and a reduction in both physical and psychological stress levels. Being supported to reconnect with your authentic self and clear the clutter of the past paves the way for clarity and empowerment to make change. One word of caution: do not make life-changing decisions in haste as hormone fluctuations can be volatile.

SELF-HELP TECHNIQUES

The ability to do something positive for yourself is particularly important during menopause when some aspects of health and wellness can seem out of your control. Being able to restore balance and ground yourself in the moment can alter the course of the day. Developing a regular practice can have very positive benefits for both physical and emotional health, improving mood and sleep patterns, which can both be detrimentally affected during menopause.

If you can rest or exercise outside, all the better. Exercise is known to promote feel-good chemicals in the brain called endorphins that improve mood levels (see also Chapter 5); while research proves that access to green space is associated with better health and wellness, including reductions in levels of stress and anxiety, improved mood, feelings of calm, and less mental fatigue. So why not try gentle movement such as yoga (see also page 186) or t'ai chi outside—both are known to be nurturing for body, mind, and spirit.

CHOOSE THE BEST EXERCISES FOR YOU

Breathing is vital to life, so it makes sense to harness the power of the breath to help control stress levels and improve mental

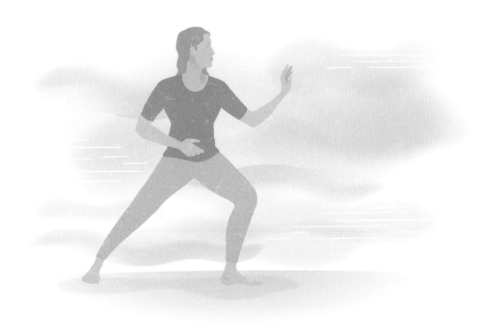

" "

The way that you choose to navigate your menopause transition
will be unique to you. Give yourself permission to take some
time to rest, reflect, and restore to enable you to fully
embrace the potential of every single day.

wellness. Working with the breath is the ideal place to start to support your mental health. Spending just a few minutes every day focusing on your breath can be life-changing. See also pages 91–93.

- **Mindfulness** is simply tuning in. It is about being fully present and totally engaged in the moment without allowing yourself to become distracted or to judge yourself if you do. Mindfulness is something that everyone can do, and with a little practice you will be able to bring awareness and care to every part of your being, which ultimately offers you choice for how you respond to the events and people that are part of it. See also pages 94–99.

- **Body scanning** can be a particularly useful practice for checking in to see where you are holding physical stress in your body. Simply by sitting or lying still and bringing attention to each part of your body in turn you can identify where you are holding the physical manifestations of stress. Once the area has been identified, it's important to be able to focus your attention on relieving that physical stress by focusing on each individual part of your body and relaxing it deeply. Body scanning can also be a good way to relieve negative feelings you may have about parts of your body. See also pages 100–103.

- **Journaling** is a very helpful way to record and reflect on your thoughts and feelings. Writing your thoughts down helps keep them from going around and around in your head. Reflecting on what you have written can help you see things more clearly and with a new perspective. Ultimately, writing down your thoughts and feelings can help you identify a new way forward, reduce stress, and take back control. It can also help you recognize and appreciate the good things about your body and your life. See also pages 104–107.

- **Visualization**—or positive mental rehearsal—is a powerful way of creating a mental image of a future event. If you can visualize your goal or desire, then you can begin to see and feel what it would be like to achieve it. Creating a written or visual representation can be a very helpful way of revealing the detail of your desired outcome. See also pages 108–111.

COGNITIVE BEHAVIORAL THERAPY

CBT was developed for people with anxiety and depression, but recently it has been specifically adapted for women with menopausal symptoms. It is an approach that is becoming increasingly popular.

At King's College London, CBT has been developed specifically to help women with troublesome hot flashes and night sweats, during menopause and following breast cancer treatments. The CBT is typically brief, interactive, and educational, with a focus on helping people reduce anxiety (see page 114), to manage hot flashes and night sweats (see page 116), and improve sleep (see page 118). CBT also encourages you to challenge overly negative attitudes and beliefs about menopause as many still feel that menopause and hot flashes are socially taboo.

Several studies, in the UK and the Netherlands, with over 1,000 women, have shown that CBT significantly reduces the impact of hot flashes and night sweats, and has additional benefits to mood, sleep, and quality of life. Trials at Kings College London found CBT was effective when delivered in groups and in self-help formats. Women who were troubled by hot flashes who used a self-help CBT booklet had less troublesome hot flashes and better sleep, coped better with stress, and generally described having a restored sense of control. They experienced beneficial changes that extended beyond their hot flash symptoms.

USING CBT TO APPRAISE LIFE PLANS

Cognitive and behavioral strategies can help people make changes to improve well-being in general. A first step can be to look at life from a broad perspective—the things that you value (about yourself and your life in general), what you used to enjoy doing, and/or how you would like things to be in five years. Then you could gradually reengage in activities that you previously valued and enjoyed, but which might have fallen by the wayside over time. As women progress through menopause, they often say that they have started gradually to rebalance their lives, for example by making valuable time for themselves.

Being more active, getting more exercise, being more assertive in general, and doing something creative were the valued activities that women often aimed for in CBT sessions.

HOW TO USE THE EXERCISES

You can find helpful guided exercises for breathing, body scanning, mindfulness, visualization, journaling, and CBT in this chapter. All these exercises encourage you to pause and take time, sometimes to reflect and sometimes just to be, which will have both physical and psychological benefits. Supporting your mental wellness following the suggestions in the box (opposite) and regular practice of the exercises will help you feel more in control of everyday life and ultimately enhance your quality of life.

SUPPORTING YOUR MENTAL WELLNESS

BE KIND TO YOURSELF

This is key. We can be so hard on ourselves sometimes. Think about treating yourself the way that you would treat your best friend. Become your own best friend.

PREPARE FOR CHANGE

Educate yourself with factual information. Knowledge is only power if we use it to help ourselves. Taking back control can have a very positive effect on our mental health.

MAKE TIME FOR YOU

It is wonderful that you have given so much of your time to nurturing those that you care for, but you can only be good to others when you are truly good to yourself.

NOURISH YOURSELF

Consider how you are nourishing your mind, body, and soul. Take stock of how you feed yourself physically, mentally, and spiritually and make changes.

COMMUNICATE

Talking is good for us. Keep the lines of communication open with your partner, family, friends, and colleagues. The more they know, the better they can support you.

SEEK SUPPORT

We all need support at some point, and whether you decide to turn to your primary care provider, OB/GYN, or complementary practitioner, don't be afraid to reach out.

FIND YOUR TRIBE

It's so important to have people to communicate with who understand what you are going through— remember that support is out there if you need it.

REST AND REFLECT

Give yourself permission to take time to reflect on what has gone before and what you would like your future to look like. Plan for the time ahead.

RENEW

Giving yourself time to reflect will allow you to move forward in whatever direction you choose, either to fulfill ambitions and desires or simply to live the life that's right for you now.

WELLNESS PRACTICES

When you are able to think, feel, act, and respond in ways that have positive impacts, it allows you to enjoy a greater quality of life. Menopause is the perfect time to use some of the practices on the following pages—such as mindfulness, journaling, and visualization—as they will help you relieve stress and anxiety and offer greater balance and clarity so that you can live your life to the fullest.

WHAT YOU NEED

To pursue optimum mental wellness you need an open mind, courage, and a willingness to try new things such as body scanning, focused breathing, or mindful walking. For many of the exercises it is helpful to have a quiet space where you won't be disturbed, and for journaling or making a vision board you will need some materials.

HOW TO FOLLOW THE EXERCISES

In the following pages you will find easy-to-follow exercises and suggestions that can set you on the path to better mental wellness. There are no set rules for how you engage with the exercises, just choose one that you would like to try and follow the simple steps. You might also like to record the steps for the body scanning, breathing, and visualization practices to allow you to relax completely. This can be very useful when choosing practices that can aid sleep or help reduce anxiety. Once you have tried the exercises, you may decide to create a regular practice, combining some of them on a daily basis to maintain a sense of calm and control.

DEVELOPING YOUR PRACTICE

If you would like to learn more about a practice, you can join a class or download an app. Alternatively, you may decide the time is right to seek support from a well-being professional; if you do, please ensure that they are suitably qualified to offer support.

BREATHING BY NUMBERS

EASES ANXIETY I BOOSTS AND BALANCES MOOD I CALMS

You have to breathe, which is why it makes sense to harness the power of the breath to calm and ground you. Menopause can be a challenging time, particularly if anxiety levels have increased as a result of hormone fluctuations, but managing your breathing can help reduce anxiety quickly and simply.

Every time you breathe in you activate the sympathetic nervous system, which is connected with your fight, flight, or freeze response. When you breathe out you activate the parasympathetic nervous system, often called rest and digest, which relaxes you. Essentially, when you breathe in you tense up, and when you breathe out you relax. So, if during every breath cycle you breathe out for a little longer than you breathe in, you are much more likely to relax. In addition, if you count each cycle of in and out breath, you engage with the rational part of your brain too, resulting in a calmer, more relaxed you. With a little practice you can learn to take back control of your thinking, allowing you to calm down and reduce stress levels, which is a vital tool for life.

COUNT YOUR BREATHS

1

Find a quiet place where you won't be disturbed and lie down or sit with your legs uncrossed. Close your eyes and become aware of your feet resting on the floor and your body touching the floor or chair.

2

Take a deep breath in for a count of three and then gently breathe out for a count of five. Continue breathing in for a count of three and out for a count of five. Notice how as you breathe out you relax.

3

Continue for a few minutes, relaxing body and mind. When ready, open your eyes and continue with your day, knowing that you now have the power to relax and take back control whenever you need to.

COLOR BREATHING

IMPROVES SLEEP I EASES ANXIETY I REDUCES TENSION

Good-quality sleep is vital for physical and mental health and well-being. This is never more important than during the menopause transition. Many women find that changes in their sleep patterns can be one of the first indications that they are experiencing the hormonal fluctuations of perimenopause.

Insomnia is a very common problem during menopause, and can be quite debilitating. Going to bed and not being able to get to sleep, or going to sleep and then lying awake in the early hours of the morning can be very distressing and leave you feeling tired and lacking in energy.

If your sleep is continually disturbed, it's important to seek professional advice, but there are also steps that you can take to help yourself. A good sleep routine and the right environment is key to helping enjoy good-quality, restful sleep, and ending the day in a calm state of mind is vital.

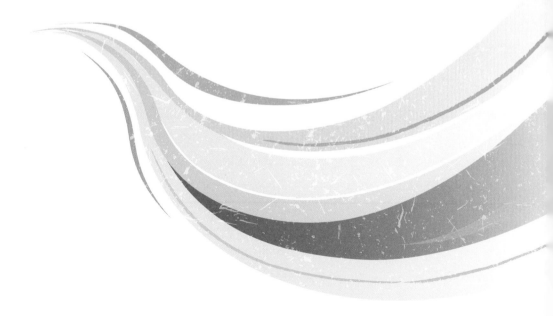

COLOR IN, COLOR OUT

1

Make sure your bedroom is as dark as possible and do not have your phone or other devices with you in your bedroom. Lie down comfortably in bed.

2

Close your eyes and bring your attention to your breath. If other thoughts come to mind, just gently refocus and bring your attention back to your breath.

3

Place your hands on your stomach and let your elbows rest gently by your side. Notice how your stomach rises and falls as you gently breathe in and breathe out.

4

Breathe in and out slowly and deeply, ensuring that your out breath is just a little longer than your in breath. Focus on this pattern for a few minutes.

5

As your breathing pattern slows to a pace that feels comfortable, visualize the breath coming into your nose and out of your mouth as your favorite restful color.

6

As you continue to breathe slowly and deeply, become aware of breathing your favorite restful color in through your nose and back out of your mouth.

7

Every time you breathe in, visualize that restful breath moving all through your body as you settle deeper and deeper into the support of the bed.

8

As you breathe out, watch the physical and mental stresses of the day float away on your restful breath, allowing the mind to clear and the body to relax.

9

Continue bringing your awareness to the breath as you relax both body and mind, which will allow you to drift peacefully into a truly restful sleep.

MINUTE MINDFULNESS

EASES ANXIETY I BOOSTS MOOD I IMPROVES SLEEP I AIDS CONCENTRATION

Mindfulness is essentially tuning in; it is simply being present and noticing thoughts, physical sensations, and senses. You can be mindful every day in everything that you do. This useful exercise will become your go-to practice during menopause; it can be used any time, anywhere, to restore equilibrium.

You may often find yourself multitasking, doing one thing while thinking about several other things—this is the opposite of mindfulness. Being mindful involves being 100 percent in the moment.

While a formal, seated mindfulness practice can be very nourishing, not everybody feels that they can commit to that time or effort, particularly during menopause when many of the symptoms make it difficult for you to settle either physically or mentally. The following

practice allows you to have brief moments of mindfulness throughout your day, so is an ideal place to start.

By following this exercise and tuning into your body several times every day, you will be able to fully notice and appreciate physical sensations and emotions. As this becomes part of your daily practice, you will find that the cumulative effect of stopping and tuning in for just one minute at a time can have a powerful impact on how you think, feel, act, and respond.

“ ”

No one is too busy to take just one minute to improve their mental wellness. Giving yourself permission to be mindful for just one minute can make all the difference in helping you change your mindset and ultimately change your life.

REST AND RESTORE

1

Choose a morning activity where you can spend one minute being mindful, for example while brushing your teeth. Appreciate the sights, sounds, smells, tastes, and feel.

2

Have a mindful breakfast. Many people are rushing in the morning, so sit and notice the smell, textures, flavors, and temperature of the food you are eating.

3

Bring just one minute of mindfulness to your work—remember you are simply tuning in. If you find it helps you concentrate, try extending your minute to two or five minutes.

4

Whatever you are doing during the day, do at least one minute of it mindfully. If your mind wanders, without judgment bring it back to the task.

5

Spend one minute outside at the end of the day, allowing the sights and sounds to come and go. It could be as simple as feeling the sun or rain on you.

6

Mindful breathing is the perfect way to end the day. When you are in bed, bring your awareness to your breath and enjoy the feeling of the breath.

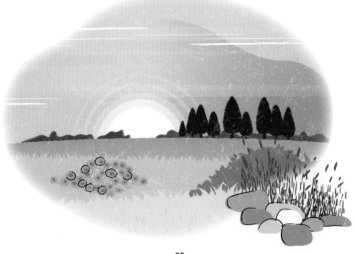

MINDFUL WALKING

BOOSTS MOOD I REENERGIZES I CALMS I IMPROVES SLEEP

Walking is good for us. It can improve our physical health as well as boosting our mental health—and best of all, it's free. Exercise can be challenging for some, particularly during menopause, so mindful walking can be the perfect solution to getting gentle exercise, improving mood, and reducing stress levels.

Our busy lives can mean that we rush from place to place without appreciating the wonder of the body that conveys us, or the sights, sounds, and aromas. You probably walk every day and pay little attention either to the sensation of walking or to what is going on around you. Mindful walking is an ideal introduction to mindfulness as it fits so beautifully into our everyday activities. This is the perfect opportunity to truly experience life, the sensation of walking and connection with the senses rather than being lost in our thoughts or engrossed in our phones. You might just be surprised by what you notice when you walk mindfully and the benefits you will gain.

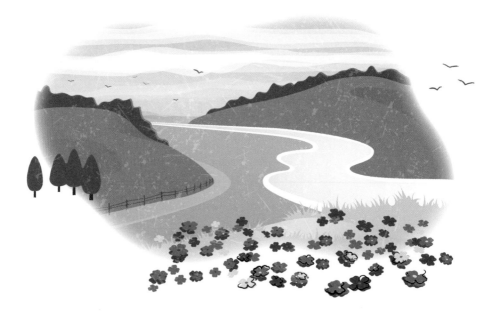

EXPLORE YOUR SENSES

1

Find a peaceful outdoor space to walk in—being in a park or forest, or by a river or the sea is ideal if you are fortunate enough to live near these locations.

2

Begin by simply noticing your feet and how they feel as they come into contact with—and then leave—the ground with each step. Simply observe the sensations.

3

Gently bring your attention to what you can see: the people, animals, birds, colors, shapes, etc. There is no need to actively think about them; just observe them.

4

Become aware of the sounds around you for a few minutes; just allow the sounds to gently come into your awareness. There is no need to label them; just notice them.

5

If you notice your mind wandering at any point, without judgment, simply return your awareness to your feet as they come into contact with the ground.

6

For a few minutes bring your attention to your sense of smell. Just allow yourself to notice the different aromas as they come and go, in and out of your nostrils.

7

Bring your awareness to all your senses, allowing the sights, sounds, and smells to simply come and go. Enjoy the sensation of being fully connected to your senses.

8

Gently bring your awareness back to your feet as they touch the ground with each step. Simply acknowledge the sensation of your feet on the ground.

9

As you come to the end of your mindful walk, take a moment to pause and consider how you might take this mindful awareness with you into the remainder of your day.

USING TECH MINDFULLY

EASES ANXIETY | BOOSTS MOOD | IMPROVES SLEEP | AIDS CONCENTRATION

Technology has become such a major part of our lives that few of us now question it. Using technology mindfully during perimenopause and menopause ensures that it remains a useful and valuable tool rather than something that detrimentally controls us and our time.

Before you pick up your phone or any other device, ask yourself why you are picking it up; what is your intention? Are you using it to make an important call or to respond to an urgent email, or are you picking it up simply out of habit?

Many women turn to social media during menopause for support—and this can be very helpful—but mindlessly scrolling through negative posts can quickly become overwhelming. The key to using technology mindfully is to choose what you have loaded onto your devices, carefully select who you follow or interact with, always know why you are using your device, and pre-set boundaries. You have a choice about how to use technology; choose wisely for your mental health and wellness.

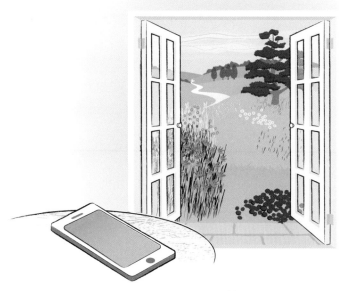

DEVICE DETOX

1
Before you pick up your device, stop, breathe, and examine your reason for using technology. Knowing why you are using your device allows you to remain mindful.

2
Decide on a time limit for interaction with your devices. It is very easy for time to slide by when mindlessly scrolling, but predefining a time limit will keep you focused.

3
Regularly clean up your emails, unsubscribe from apps that you don't use, and unfollow people or pages that you don't find supportive, helpful, or positive.

4
Notifications or alerts are essentially there to prompt you to check your phone every time they go off. A simple way to control this is to turn them off and take back control.

5
If you find yourself mindlessly checking your email on your phone many times a day, delete it. Set times to check your email on a device that is not always with you.

6
When eating, put your phone away. Constant interruptions from technology can stop you from both mindfully eating your food and connecting with those around you.

7
Turn off all your devices at least an hour before you plan to go to bed. This will help you truly turn off and will help ensure a more restful night's sleep.

8
Choose a day to go tech free. Set your intention to have 24 hours free from any screens and see how it feels. Instead, take a mindful walk or enjoy a creative hobby.

9
Holidays should be a change from routine— time to rest, relax, and restore. Take a digital vacation so you can disconnect physically and mentally and improve well-being.

BODY APPRECIATION SCAN

INCREASES SELF-ESTEEM I BOOSTS MOOD I MAY IMPROVE LIBIDO

We rarely take the time to appreciate our bodies and how truly amazing they are. Menopause can bring challenges when your body starts to change and both act and react in ways that you are not accustomed to. This body scan will help you confidently accept your changing body.

Taking the time to appreciate and show gratitude for the wonder of your body not only brings your attention to so much that you may take for granted, but also brings you a deeper connection and acceptance for the body that will carry you from perimenopause through post-menopause. It can improve self-esteem, mood, and libido.

This body scan will allow you to tune in and connect with all the parts of your body as you bring your attention to each part in turn. If you feel discomfort or judgment about a particular part of your body during the exercise, hold one hand over your heart and the other hand over that part of your body and visualize sending loving kindness.

Women experiencing menopause at an early age or due to medical treatment will particularly benefit from engaging in a body scan as it can enhance self-compassion.

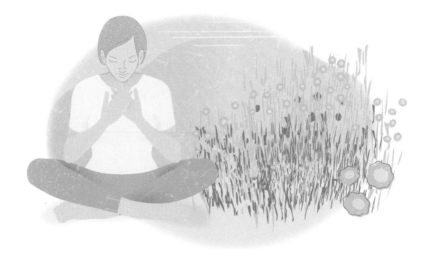

ACCEPT AND APPRECIATE

1
Settle yourself comfortably, sitting or lying down. Bring your attention to your breath and feel the rise and fall of your body as you breathe in and breathe out.

2
Once settled, begin by considering your nose and mouth. Appreciate the functions that they perform all day every day, allowing you to breathe, to smell, and to taste.

3
Gently bring your attention to your eyes and ears. Consider how important they are to you every day of your life—how they allow you to see and hear the ones you love.

4
Consider your brain and how vital it is to every waking and sleeping moment; how it is the most incredible organ. Bring appreciation and gratitude to your brain.

5
Move your attention to your spine and take time to appreciate the complexity of the vital central support structure that carries your neck and head so effortlessly.

6
Bring appreciation to your arms, hands, legs, and feet. Then turn your attention to your torso, to the vulva and vagina, and the organs of the pelvis and send loving kindness.

7
Bring your focus to your lungs and back to the breath and take a moment to appreciate the wonder of your lungs and the function that they perform.

8
Place your hands over your heart and send thanks for the magnificence of your heart. Appreciate the wonder of your body, how it supports you.

9
Visualize appreciation and gratitude flowing to every part of your unique body, then let your focus return to your breath. Slowly open your eyes to end.

BODY SCAN FOR INSOMNIA

EASES ANXIETY I IMPROVES SLEEP I CALMS I REDUCES TENSION

One of the most troublesome menopausal symptoms for many women can be insomnia. If you are struggling to get to sleep at night, or are waking during the early hours of the morning and find that you just can't get back to sleep, this body scan exercise can help.

There is nothing worse than lying awake, just wishing you could go back to sleep. Unfortunately, the result of this is often increased anxiety, tension, and a busy mind—so having something that you can do to help yourself is important.

Body scanning using progressive muscle relaxation can help relax body and mind and relieve tension, so it is ideal for use during menopause. During this exercise as you work your way around the body you will be tensing individual muscle groups as you breathe in, then slowly relaxing them to release tension as you breathe out. Notice how it feels for the muscles to be tense and how it feels for them to be truly relaxed.

A good night's sleep is critical to good health and can have a significant impact on your energy levels, concentration, and mental health. Many women find that sleep can be an issue during menopause, either struggling to go to sleep or waking often in the night, so it's important to be able to use techniques such as this relaxing body scan to help you enter the sleep phase and enjoy a truly restful night's sleep.

Sleep should be considered as vital as the air that we breathe; it is key to physical health and mental wellness. When hormones start to fluctuate during perimenopause, sleep can be disrupted. Recognize that this is not your fault—be kind to yourself and rest when you need to.

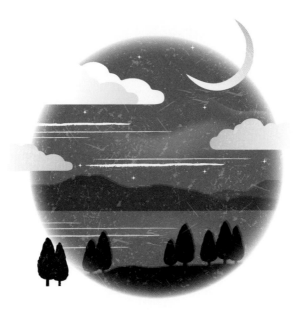

RELEASE THE TENSION

1

Lie comfortably on your back, then focus purely on your breath. Starting with your left foot, breathe in and tense your left foot and lower leg.

2

Hold the tension for a few seconds, and then as you breathe out allow your left leg to relax. Tense and release the thigh muscles in your left leg.

3

Do the same on your right leg, starting with the feet and working up to the thigh. Tense and relax the muscles as you slowly breathe in and out.

4

Breathe in and out as you tense and relax the muscles around your body: first your buttocks, then your stomach muscles, and then your back.

5

Shrug your shoulders up toward your ears to tense, then relax. Clench and relax your neck and your biceps. Make your hands into fists, then release.

6

Frown hard, then relax your forehead. Squeeze your eyes shut and tense your cheeks, then relax. Squeeze your lips together, then smile.

WORRY JOURNAL

CALMS I BOOSTS MOOD I AIDS CONCENTRATION I IMPROVES SLEEP

You can lose hours worrying … possibly even days. Worry is essentially a misuse of the imagination, which can lead to stress. During menopause, worry can take on a whole new dimension, particularly if you don't recognize what's happening to you or if symptoms are having a detrimental effect on your overall health.

Worries can be like laundry going around and around in the washing machine of the mind, so it's important to empty the machine from time to time and put those worries into perspective, as you would sort out your laundry. Writing your worries down can be a powerful way of ensuring that they don't become bigger than they really are, when they will start to interfere with your sleep and increase your stress levels.

We all cope differently with change, and during menopause things are changing for many women. Unexpected change can lead to worry and increased levels of stress and anxiety. When stress and anxiety become overwhelming it can feel paralyzing, so having a simple tool that you can use to examine those worries on a daily basis can be crucial. By following these simple steps you can learn to take control of your worries.

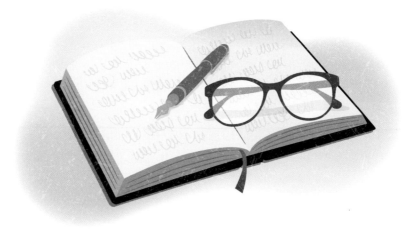

RECORD AND RELEASE

1

Decide where you will record your worries—choose something that you can keep with you at all times. A small, pocket-sized paper journal is ideal, or you can use your phone.

2

Every time a new worry appears, write it down right away and make the active choice to leave it in your worry journal until you are ready to consider it later.

3

Schedule 15 minutes at the same time every day—ideally later in the day but not too near bedtime—to consider any worries that are written in your worry journal.

4

Before you open your worry journal, center yourself by focusing on your breath for two minutes. Simply notice the breath coming into your nose and out of your mouth.

5

During your worry time consider each of the worries in your journal in turn and ask yourself how anxious each is making you feel on a scale from 1 to 10.

6

Ask yourself what evidence you have for the worry. Is it real or is it imagined? If you decide it is imagined, recognize it for the story that it is and let the worry go.

7

If you decide the worry is real, ask yourself: can I take action to alleviate the worry today? If the answer is yes, do it—take the action and diffuse the worry.

8

If you recognize that you can't do anything about the worry, leave it in the book for another day. Scale each worry again and notice if you are feeling differently about it.

9

Once you have considered each worry, close the journal and put it away until the next time you need to record a worry. Appreciate that the worry washing is done.

GRATITUDE JOURNAL

EASES ANXIETY I BOOSTS MOOD I IMPROVES CONFIDENCE I EVOKES JOY

Keeping a gratitude journal has become increasingly popular over the past few years, and while it can be an enjoyable thing to do, studies have also shown that there are real health benefits to be gained. Focusing on all the good things in your life during menopause is nourishing for your mind, body, and spirit.

Gratitude journaling can be a really helpful practice during menopause, especially if you are not feeling particularly grateful for some of the unpleasant symptoms you might be experiencing.

The wonderful thing about writing down your thoughts is that it helps you organize them and put them into some sort of perspective, and allows you to reflect upon their emotional impact. To make the most of this powerful tool, try to write your journal once a week using the prompts opposite. Reading your gratitude journal can be a great source of hope and joy on days that are proving challenging.

In addition to your weekly journal, end each day by asking yourself this question: "What's the best thing that happened to me today?" There will always be something.

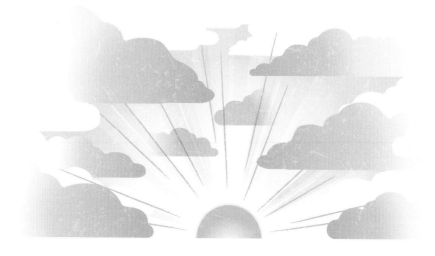

FIVE BLESSINGS

1

Take some time to choose your journal. Make it a book that you want to pick up every week. It can be purchased or homemade, but make it special to you.

2

Give yourself permission to schedule time once every week to write in your journal. Diarizing it allows you to acknowledge and value yourself.

3

Before you sit down to write, choose a favorite pen or pencil, ensure you won't be disturbed, make yourself a soothing drink, and turn off your phone.

4

Settle down comfortably and allow yourself plenty of time. Consider just five things that you are grateful for and focus on the detail of each one.

5

If you are struggling to find five positive things, concentrate on the simple things you may take for granted. Shelter, clean water, nature, and loved ones are all good examples.

6

Take time to consider just what each one of the five blessings you have chosen means to you and what really matters in your life and write it down in your journal.

❝ ❞

Never underestimate the power of offering silent thanks for the little things that matter, as together those little things create the vibration of our lives and can help make the menopause transition infinitely easier to manage.

BOOSTING CONFIDENCE

IMPROVES CONFIDENCE I INCREASES SELF-ESTEEM I BOOSTS MOOD

Self-confidence tends to make us feel happier, and when we feel happier we are less likely to be fearful of tackling future challenges as we have positive experiences in the past to support us. This can help us embrace the future, take action, and achieve our goals during menopause and beyond.

During menopause many women report that they feel they are losing their confidence. We all have different levels of self-confidence, and loss of confidence can often be directly linked to hormone fluctuations during perimenopause and menopause.

Studies show that thoughts can be as powerful as actions, and visualizations or positive mental rehearsal has proven to be very effective in helping people achieve their dreams. Menopause is often described as the third stage of a woman's life, and historically women entering this stage were referred to as "wise women" due to the life experience that they carried with them. Seeking professional support to help you explore any issues that you feel could be holding you back from feeling more confident can be very helpful, but it's also important to have some tools to be able to improve things yourself and to allow you to channel your own inner wise woman. Menopause can be the ideal time to reflect on your past successes in order to inform your future. The following exercise will help you do exactly that.

" "

Stop waiting for confidence to arrive—confidence comes with experience. Finding the courage to express your authentic self without the burden of comparison or trying to be perfect will allow the world to benefit from everything you bring and see you shine in all your unique glory.

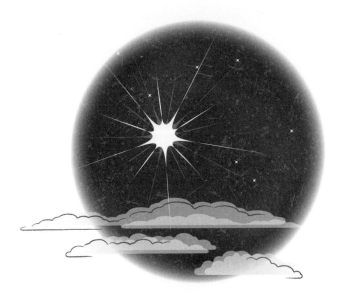

BE THE STAR

1

Think about when you have felt particularly confident in the past. This will remind you that you can feel this way even if it's not how you feel now.

2

Focus on one situation where you would like to feel more confident—it could be a meeting or a social event. Write down how you would ideally experience it.

3

Think about the event and imagine that everything works out perfectly. How would you like to feel? What would you like to see and hear?

4

Close your eyes and imagine that you are playing the starring role in a film of the event, successfully accomplishing your goal as you planned.

5

Practice visualizing this positive situation. By doing this visualization every day you can perfect your performance to ensure success in the future.

6

Pick a positive affirmation that describes how confident you feel about achieving your goal and say it out loud every day.

LOOKING TO THE FUTURE

CALMS I BOOSTS MOOD I IMPROVES CONFIDENCE I EVOKES JOY

Menopause can be a time of transition and ultimately transformation which, for many, includes consideration of how they would like their future to be. Giving yourself the time to consider possibilities and work toward fulfilling long-held dreams and ambitions can be a very enjoyable and empowering exercise.

Once you have brought together all the pieces of the puzzle, it can be helpful to create a vision board that represents your ideal future. Visualization is a powerful tool in helping to make that vision a reality.

A word of caution: menopause can be transformational in many ways. For some this can include a complete spring cleaning of some or all aspects of their lives. While this can be freeing, it can also feel overwhelming and might be the ideal time to seek some professional support. Whether you decide to consider the future with or without this support, remember to take your time. Don't make decisions in haste—this is the rest of your life, and it matters.

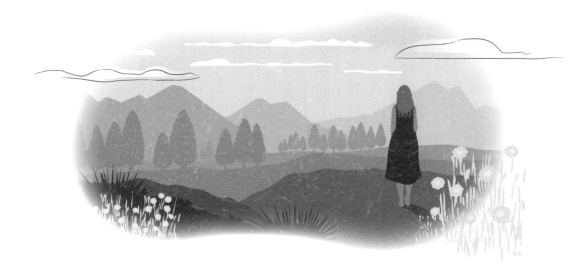

CREATE YOUR VISION

1

Sit quietly and consider the major areas of your life. This could include work, relationships, health, finances, and personal development. How do they look now?

2

Ask yourself, if you could wave a magic wand what would life look like in the future? Consider how you would like each area of your life to be and write it down in detail.

3

Think about what is important to you and form a clear vision of how you would like your future life to be. Create a visual representation of that life—a vision board.

4

Creating a vision board can be a very enjoyable thing to do. Either make it on your computer and print it out, or stick images from magazines onto a piece of cardboard.

5

Once you are satisfied that your vision board represents everything you are aiming for, put it up where you can see it every day to remind you what you are aiming for.

6

Now it's time to consider the steps you will need to take to move you closer to your ideal future. Remember that hard work, perseverance, and time are key here.

7

Sit quietly every day and visualize the future life that you want to move toward. See yourself taking the steps you need, and overcoming challenges.

8

Allow yourself to imagine what it would feel like to achieve your goals. What would you be doing? Who would you be spending time with?

9

Don't forget to celebrate every little step toward achieving your aim. Every step will take you further along the path to your vision of the future.

COGNITIVE BEHAVIORAL THERAPY (CBT)

CBT is a nonmedical approach that encourages you to understand the links between thoughts (cognitions), emotions, physical reactions, and behavior. It helps you develop practical ways to manage stress and provides coping skills and useful strategies to improve well-being. It is becoming increasingly popular to help with menopausal symptoms such as anxiety, hot flashes, and insomnia.

HOW TO FOLLOW CBT PRACTICES

CBT follows structured sessions, and between sessions you are encouraged to complete homework tasks, trying out practical coping strategies in your daily life and then discussing how they worked.

During CBT sessions you will be helped to work through a typical negative cycle that can apply for hot flashes, stress, anxiety, low mood, or sleep problems (see opposite), recognizing how your cognitive and behavioral reactions can exacerbate the problem. You will then be shown how to use CBT techniques and strategies to help break the cycle. You can either see a CBT counselor, participate in a group session, or use the self-help exercises that follow (see pages 114–119).

HOW TO ACCESS CBT

CBT is widely available with psychologists, social workers and therapists. You can also get more information and look for a therapist at the National Association of Cognitive Behavioral therapists: www.nacbt.org.

There are also useful CBT fact sheets for women and for health professionals and self-help books that specifically cover CBT practices for menopause (see page 219).

CYCLE OF THOUGHTS AND BEHAVIORAL REACTIONS

Negative situations that cause hot flashes, anxiety, low mood, and sleep problems.

Alternative ways to think and react that are compassionate and more neutral.

NEGATIVE CYCLE

APPLYING CBT

BEHAVIOR
Avoid situations, do less, eat or drink too much, stay in bed or nap during the day.

BEHAVIOR
Use calm breathing, try to continue with activities, eat well, exercise, try not to nap.

PHYSICAL SYMPTOMS
Hot, sweating, tense, tired, palpitations, headache.

PHYSICAL SYMPTOMS
Hot, sweating, tense, tired, palpitations, headache.

THOUGHTS
My body is out of control! I'm not good enough. I'll never get back to sleep.

THOUGHTS
I will feel calmer if I relax. I shouldn't assume I know what people think about me. It's normal to wake up during the night.

FEELINGS
Frustrated, hopeless, embarrassed, sad, and anxious.

FEELINGS
Calm, hopeful, accepting, neutral, confident.

Adapted from Women's Health Concern
CBT Factsheet (see page 219).

CBT FOR ANXIETY

EASES ANXIETY I CALMS I BOOSTS MOOD I REDUCES TENSION

CBT was developed for people with anxiety and depression, and it is considered to be an effective treatment for these problems. Because midlife is a time when many women are juggling multiple demands with little time for themselves, as well as negative attitudes toward menopause, CBT can be very beneficial.

How you experience menopause is affected by your attitudes and expectations about menopause and aging, and by what is happening in your life, as well as by your hormones. For example, if you feel stressed at work or at home and have too many demands, and at the same time feel that you are entering a stage of life where you will become invisible, considered of lesser value, or be ridiculed, not surprisingly you might feel low in mood or anxious. In addition, anxiety, low mood, hot flashes, and sleep problems can all interact in a vicious cycle.

HOW CBT CAN HELP
CBT strategies aim to intervene and break these negative cycles and to alleviate the physical and the psychological symptoms that can occur during menopause. Research shows that CBT seems to work by changing how women think about menopause and about symptoms, as well as providing helpful cognitive and behavioral strategies. By adopting these strategies, you can be more accepting of menopause and its changes, which will allow you to cope more calmly with any stresses or worries.

Writing down your thoughts, feelings, and behavioral reactions can help you understand how and what you are feeling (see opposite). You can then use CBT techniques to develop practical ways to manage problems by using new coping skills and useful strategies.

66 99

Anxiety often increases during menopause, and having a way to cope with stress and worry is essential. CBT will help you find kinder, more supportive alternatives to any negative thoughts you may be having.

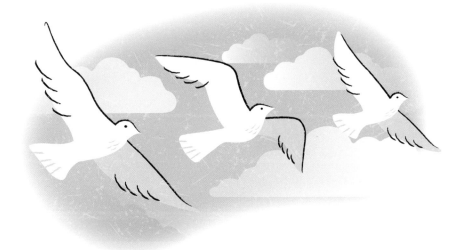

REFRAME UNHELPFUL THOUGHTS

1
Choose a quiet spot where you won't be disturbed and have a paper and pen at hand. Think of a time when you have felt stressed or anxious. Try to remember that situation clearly.

2
Write down what physical symptoms or sensations you were aware of when you were experiencing that situation, for example tense shoulders, sweating, or heart palpitations.

3
Ask yourself how you felt when you were in that situation. You are looking for emotions such as embarrassment, frustration, or anger. Write down these emotions under "feelings."

4
Write down your "behaviors"—what you do when you feel like this. Ask yourself what is going through your mind when you have these feelings.

5
Think about whether your thoughts and behavioral reactions are helpful; and if not; consider what would be more supportive reactions.

6
Apply this to all areas of life. For example, if you are worried you "can't cope at work," instead think, "I have managed before, so I know I can do it."

CBT FOR HOT FLASHES

REDUCES NIGHT SWEATS | SOOTHES FLUSHED SKIN | REDUCES PALPITATIONS

Hot flashes and night sweats are two of the main physical symptoms that many women experience during menopause. CBT helps you identify the key thoughts that you have during a hot flash, so that you can calmly accept them. Being anxious and stressed can make hot flashes even more problematic.

One of the key messages of CBT is that your perspective within situations influences how you feel and how you will cope. For example, if you have a hot flash at work and worry your colleagues will tease you, you are likely to feel embarrassed and more anxious. These emotional reactions can increase physical arousal, which intensifies the hot flash.

BREAKING THE CYCLE

CBT aims to break the negative hot flash cycle, changing how you think about hot flashes and using behavioral strategies, such as calm abdominal breathing (see opposite) to help you cope with them. CBT also helps you discover and write down possible triggers—such as coffee, alcohol, spicy foods, and stress—so that you can try to avoid or control them.

MANAGING A HOT FLASH

Using CBT techniques can help you identify and document the key thoughts that you experience while having a hot flash (see also page 88).

First, consider whether that thought is helpful or not and how it makes you feel. Then find an alternative way to think and react that is compassionate and more neutral. By accepting the symptoms and not reacting with frustration or anxiety, you may find that hot flashes are easier to cope with in your everyday life.

❝ ❞

CBT encourages you to challenge social taboos and overly negative attitudes and beliefs about menopause and symptoms such as hot flashes and night sweats.

ABDOMINAL BREATHING

1

Lie down comfortably and just follow your breath with your attention. Keep your chest and shoulders still and push your stomach out as you breathe in. Place one hand on your chest and one hand on your stomach.

2

Keep the hand on your chest fairly still—the hand on your stomach should rise and fall. Relax your shoulders and just focus on your breathing for a few minutes. This can give you time to think about how to react in a stressful situation.

3

Once familiar with abdominal breathing, you can use it at the onset of a hot flash or night sweat, as well as to help you in stressful situations and to calm you if you find that you are struggling to get to sleep (see page 118).

CBT FOR SLEEP

IMPROVES SLEEP | REDUCES NIGHT SWEATS | CALMS RESTLESS LEGS

During the menopause transition, sleep can often be broken by night sweats; and anxiety, stress, and low mood can interfere with the amount of sleep you have, as well as its quality. But there are various strategies you can use to help improve your sleep, and therefore your overall well-being.

CBT can help you identify and change thoughts and actions that can cause or exacerbate sleep problems. First, spend some time considering what may be worrying you and disrupting your sleep. Maybe write down your concerns or list them in your phone, identifying any worries you have about sleep or night sweats (see also page 114). Work out ways you can help yourself get back to sleep, whether by focusing on muscle relaxation techniques or abdominal breathing (see page 117). If you practice these during the day, you will find that they are easier to use at night.

Next, take time to look at your routine and what changes you can make. Behavioral strategies you can put in place include keeping regular times to go to bed and get up in the mornings and avoiding sleeping late or having naps. Having a wind-down time—when you relax an hour or so before bedtime—and getting exercise earlier in the day are helpful, too.

NIGHT SWEATS

Night sweats are a common menopausal symptom but can severely disrupt sleep, leading to fatigue. Manage night sweats using breathing, calm thoughts, and an automatic routine to cool down. Get up, cool your body down, and calm your thoughts, as stress can make it harder to get back to sleep. Then get back into bed and focus on abdominal breathing.

❝ ❞

As with hot flashes during the day, the key to managing night sweats is to use cognitive behavioral strategies to remain calm. Feeling anxious about missed sleep just makes it more difficult to get back to sleep.

GOOD SLEEP HYGIENE

1

Make sure that you have an established calming routine at bedtime. Take time to have a bath or read a book before you go to bed. Creating good habits will help you train your body's natural rhythms to facilitate sleep.

2

Create a calm and tranquil haven for you to sleep in. Make sure that your bedroom isn't too hot, and you have light sleepwear. Keep all electronics out of the bedroom, and turn your mobile phone off at least an hour before bed.

3

Address any stress or worrying thoughts you may be experiencing. Use abdominal breathing (see page 117) to calm you and to help you either get to sleep or get back to sleep if you have been woken up by a hot flash.

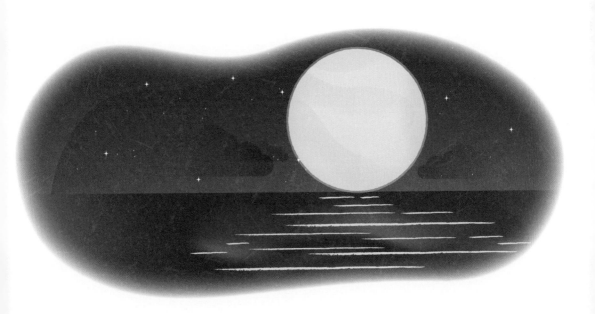

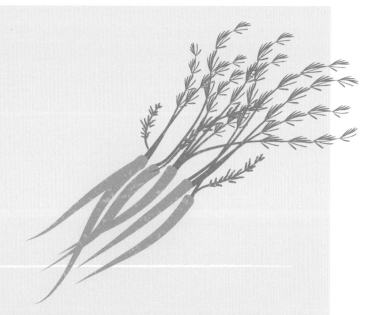

NUTRITION

INTRODUCTION

As your body changes during perimenopause and menopause, so do your dietary needs. A well-balanced diet is essential because it enables your body to adjust to hormonal changes and is critical to maintaining good bone, brain, heart, liver, and gut health, as well as managing many common menopausal symptoms.

It is important to evaluate your diet because optimum nutrition during menopause will provide you with a multitude of benefits. You need to eat whole foods that will provide the required nutrients necessary for a smooth transition. Good nutrition will enable you to protect your bones, maintain a healthy weight, boost your mood and energy levels, and help reduce or alleviate many menopausal symptoms.

Eating a nutrient-dense diet will supply you with all the necessary protein, healthy fats, carbohydrates, vitamins, minerals, and phytonutrients needed to ensure that your body, brain, and hormones function at their best. To do this, increase the amount of fruit and vegetables, whole grains, dairy products, seafood, lean meats, eggs, beans, seeds, and nuts in your diet.

IMPROVE BONE DENSITY

Bone density peaks in your late twenties, then starts to decline around the age of 35. The decline is exacerbated by hormonal changes at menopause, potentially leading to bone frailty and an increased risk of fractures and osteoporosis. However, a good diet and weight-bearing exercise (see Chapter 5) can help maintain bone density before, during, and after menopause, reducing the risk of osteoporosis, which currently one in two women will develop.

To maintain strong bones, ensure you have a good intake of both calcium (see page 143) and vitamin D (see page 141), as well as minerals such as zinc and magnesium (see page 144), essential fatty acids (see page 132), and collagen.

BENEFIT HEART HEALTH

There is a strong link between good nutrition and a healthy heart, which is important because menopausal hormone changes can bring increased cardiovascular risk in the form of higher blood pressure and cholesterol levels. In fact, more than half of women over 50 will die from heart disease.

Eating a rainbow of fruit and vegetables will provide you with nutrient-dense foods, as well as a wide range of heart-friendly

" "

During menopause your nutritional requirements change and you need greater fortification from foods full of vitamins and minerals in order to maintain good bone, muscle, gut, heart, and brain health.

antioxidants. In addition, consumption of green leafy vegetables and vitamin C-rich fruit and vegetables seems to have a protective effect against coronary heart disease. Essential fatty acids (see page 132) are also very beneficial for heart health.

BOOST BRAIN HEALTH

Menopause is often associated with mild cognitive changes, such as memory loss and brain fog, so it's important to eat well to maximize your brain function.

Your brain is 60 percent fat, and fats are very important for brain function. You need to eat the right kinds of "good" fats such as

omega-3 fatty acids (see page 132) to maintain brain health and good cognition. In addition, you should avoid trans or "bad" fats that make memory function and concentration less efficient. You should also boost your intake of foods rich in B vitamins (see page 140), vitamin C, and vitamin E.

IMPROVE GUT HEALTH

The gut is involved in digestion, vitamin production, and weight regulation. It kills off harmful bacteria, reduces inflammation, and controls your immune system. A healthy gut has a crucial role to play in combating conditions such as diabetes, heart disease,

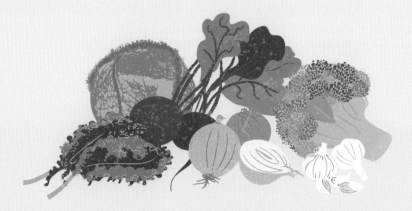

and obesity, which can become problematic during menopause. There is also evidence that good gut health may help prevent low mood and anxiety, which are often associated with menopause.

Gut health and gut bacteria are the most overlooked elements of hormonal balance. As hormone levels change during menopause, this can affect your gut health, leading to serious digestive problems, flatulence, and bloating.

The gut is home to trillions of bacteria, known as gut microbes. The gut microbiome controls the production of hormones and inhibits or supports hormonal balance. What you eat and drink has a significant effect on your gut health, so it is important to eat natural, unprocessed foods that encourage the growth of friendly gut bacteria, as well as both prebiotic and probiotic foods (see page 146).

AID LIVER HEALTH

The liver has many vital functions, including storing energy, helping maintain blood glucose levels, and cleaning and detoxifying the blood. It helps with blood clotting, stores specific vitamins, and helps synthesize your hormones. During menopause, if your liver is under stress your hormonal balance can be affected dramatically, which can exacerbate menopausal symptoms.

To boost your liver health you need to have plenty of detoxifying foods such as green leafy vegetables, citrus fruits, and herbal teas. See also page 147.

HELP WITH WEIGHT MANAGEMENT

As you get older, your metabolism naturally slows down, so to maintain the same weight you need to reduce your calorie intake. Every decade you should eat around 100 fewer calories per day; for example, a 50-year-old needs approximately 300 fewer calories than a 20-year-old.

Declining estrogen levels also affect metabolism and weight distribution changes as you hit menopause, with the added fat accumulating around the stomach.

Stress, which produces cortisol in the body, can also lead to an increase in stomach fat. However, there are a number of ways you can maximize your diet to minimize weight gain (see box, right).

A menopause-friendly diet is similar to a Mediterranean-style diet—with plenty of vegetables, fruit, whole grains, and unsaturated fats found in olive oil and nuts. It includes poultry and fish and is low in red meat and processed foods.

TIPS FOR MAINTAINING A HEALTHY WEIGHT

PROTEIN

Eat high-quality protein (see page 135) and healthy fats (see page 132) at each meal to balance blood sugar levels. Nuts, seeds, eggs, and quinoa are all high in protein.

GOOD CARBS

Eat complex carbohydrates (see page 136) rather than refined carbohydrates, e.g. brown bread or rice rather than white. These help you feel full for longer.

FIBER

Add fiber (see page 138) to meals so you feel full faster, and feel full for longer, preventing blood sugar crashes and cravings. It also keeps your gut microbiome healthy.

FRESH FOOD

Don't eat out or have takeout meals too often as they are often laden with calories. Cook from fresh instead, so you can use nutritious, well-balanced ingredients.

CUT OUT VICES

Eliminate or reduce refined carbohydrates, sugar, and bad fats (see page 130). Figure out what your food vice is and slowly reduce your intake, then eliminate it completely.

GOOD SNACKS

Swap unhealthy snacks for nutritious snacks such as nuts and seeds (see page 128), and cut back on snacking throughout the day, especially in the late afternoon and evening.

PORTION SIZE

Use a smaller plate and divide it up: a quarter of your plate should be filled with whole grains; another quarter should be protein; and half should be vegetables and salad.

TIME MEALS

Start your day with warm lemon water and a protein-packed breakfast. Have your main meal at midday, and a light dinner early in the evening, then nothing until breakfast.

GUT HEALTH

Beneficial gut bacteria affect your hunger, satiety, and fat storage hormones. Boost your intake of prebiotics and probiotics (see page 146) for a healthy gut microbiome.

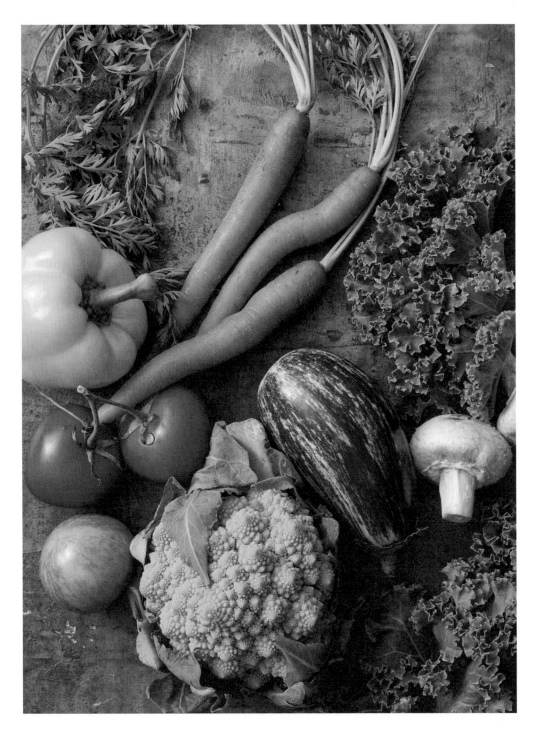

IMPROVE MOOD

Your mood can be significantly affected by blood sugar balance and hormonal imbalances. Eliminating added sugar and refined carbohydrates from your diet can lead to a marked improvement in your mood and mood fluctuations. Eating foods that are loaded with antioxidants—such as cherries, mango, and berries, as well as omega-3 fatty acids such as salmon and flax seeds (see also page 132)—can improve mood.

Plus, ensuring you have good gut health, with a high intake of fiber (see page 138), prebiotics, and probiotics (see page 146), can help improve mood and stress levels.

EAT THE RAINBOW

Increase your intake of fruit and vegetables as they are anti-aging, antioxidant, gut-boosting, nutrient-dense foods. Eating a wide variety of natural foods of every color of the rainbow every day will ensure you get the full spectrum of phytonutrients that you need to maintain optimum health.

- **Red**: peppers, tomatoes, strawberries
- **Yellow**: corn, bananas, peppers
- **Orange**: carrots, nectarines, sweet potatoes
- **Green**: broccoli, kale, edamame beans
- **Purple**: eggplant, olives, purple cabbage
- **White**: cauliflower, mushrooms, potatoes

BETTER HORMONE BALANCE

When you don't have enough protein, healthy fats, or nutrients in your diet it affects the production of hormones, putting your body under additional stress and causing hormonal imbalances. As you get older, your metabolism, which is regulated by the thyroid gland, slows down. Your thyroid is affected by a number of factors, including a poor diet, which can prevent the thyroid from getting the nutrients it needs, resulting in a slowed metabolism, increased fat storage, and generally feeling sluggish.

Phytoestrogens are plant-based compounds that mimic the effects of estrogen, and may aid hormone balance as they have the ability to occupy estrogen receptors in our bodies. Many plant-based foods contain phytoestrogens, in particular soy products and flaxseeds. There are three kinds of plant estrogens: isoflavones (in soy and legumes), lignans (in most vegetables and grains), and coumestans (in some beans and sprouted seeds). See also page 149.

Phytoestrogens are particularly beneficial during menopause because they help keep your brain and bones healthy, may help prevent certain types of cancer, and have been found to alleviate hot flashes. However, the effect of phytoestrogens on hot flashes varies between women, as only one-third to a half of women have the gut bacteria that is necessary to convert the phytoestrogens to a more potent form.

NUTRIENT-PACKED SNACKS

- Berries with a handful of nuts.
- Hummus with vegetable crudités or whole-grain crackers.
- Natural yogurt with seeds or fruit.
- A couple of squares of dark chocolate and a few almonds.
- Whole-grain pita with salsa or guacamole.

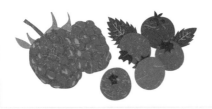

WHAT TO EAT FOR OPTIMAL HEALTH

Many women enter perimenopause or menopause with nutritional deficiencies, and this can be exacerbated by hormonal changes, so it is important to eat a balanced diet that is high in plant-based foods, and full of phytonutrients, antioxidants, vitamins, and minerals. Also consider taking nutritional supplements (see page 150).

Your body needs adequate nutrients so that your hormones can function, and be produced, stored, and transported, and this is particularly important at menopause when hormone balance is vital.

To follow The Menopause Diet (see box, opposite), make sure that your diet is full of antioxidant-rich foods such as fruits and vegetables, vitamins and minerals, gut-friendly prebiotic and probiotic foods (see page 146), as well as the key food groups.

- **Fiber** helps keep your digestive system healthy and prevent constipation, and is vital in weight management. The amount of fiber in your diet also determines how much estrogen you excrete and how much you store, making it very important during menopause. See also page 138.
- **Protein** is essential for building hormones, muscle, and healthy skin. It is particularly important for women over 40 because it is crucial for hormone balance and the metabolism of fat. Your body can't store protein, so you need a constant supply—that's why it's important to eat high-quality protein with every meal. See also page 135.
- **Good fats** are also key. Fat is high in calories; however, during menopause, it is crucial for your health, skin, and waistline, as long as you are eating the right fats in small amounts. Western diets are often deficient in the anti-inflammatory omega-3 essential fatty acids, but you need this daily as it helps lower triglycerides and improve mood, and is one of the most important nutrients for hormonal balance. See also page 132.
- **Carbohydrates** are important because they are the body's primary source of energy, plus complex carbs are nutrient-packed and contain all the essential fiber you need for healthy elimination. See also page 136.

THE MENOPAUSE DIET

STAY HYDRATED

Make sure you drink enough fluids, preferably at least eight glasses of water or herbal tea daily. You need water to keep your hormonal systems working at their best. See also page 137.

EAT REGULARLY

Don't skip meals, especially breakfast, the most important meal of the day. Have three meals a day to ensure a steady flow of energy—with a lighter meal in the early evening.

GOOD SNACKS

A healthy, protein-filled snack between meals can help keep your mood and hormone levels balanced. See box (opposite) for snacks that are packed with vitamins and minerals.

KEY FOODS

Eat high-quality protein (see page 135) at every meal. Eat the right carbs (see page 136) and good fats (see page 132), and ensure your diet is rich in fiber (see page 138).

HEALTHY GUT

Feed your good gut bacteria by boosting your intake of both prebiotic and probiotic foods (see page 146). Eat plenty of fiber to aid digestion and excretion.

PLANT-BASED

Make sure your diet is largely plant-based, with fish, good-quality poultry, or lean red meat a couple of times a week. Choose organic produce if possible.

FRUITS AND VEGETABLES

Eat a rainbow of fruits and vegetables, ideally organic—have five servings a day. Be inventive—add grated zucchini and carrots to pasta sauce or top pizzas purely with vegetables.

POWER FOODS

Boost your intake of anti-aging, antioxidant, and hormone-balancing phytoestrogen-rich foods. Plus, don't peel vegetables before cooking or eating because the skin contains antioxidants.

ELIMINATE

Reduce or cut out the following from your diet: refined sugar, caffeine, alcohol, salt, refined carbohydrates, and processed foods. See also page 130.

LOOK AT YOUR LIFESTYLE

It is important to review and alter your diet as you approach menopause so that your body is able to cope with all the hormonal changes. A better diet will also help minimize many common menopausal symptoms such as mood swings, hot flashes, and insomnia.

- **Avoid highly processed** and junk foods and prepare meals from scratch to avoid unhealthy additives and extra sugar and salt. Use herbs and spices to add flavor to food instead of using salt because too much salt can exacerbate the common menopausal issues of water retention and bloating.
- **Reduce your sugar intake** because it has been linked to numerous health problems including cancer, diabetes, and heart disease. Sugar can also overwork your liver and make it unable to process estrogen effectively, which can cause estrogen levels to fluctuate, exacerbating menopausal hormone changes. Instead of sweet foods, have healthy snacks such as nuts and olives (see also page 128).
- **Cut out "bad" saturated fats** found in many manufactured foods and increase your "good" fat intake by upping your intake of oily fish, nuts, and seeds such as flaxseeds and chia seeds.
- **Eliminate caffeine**—a natural stimulant that works by stimulating the brain and central nervous system. Drinking too much causes excess cortisol to be released into the bloodstream, which can weaken your adrenals, deplete your body of nutrients, and interfere with hormonal balance and sleep. Wean yourself off slowly and replace with lemon water or herbal teas.
- **Cut out alcohol**, which is high in calories and plays havoc with hormonal balance. It interferes with the liver's functioning and makes it less able to clear out excess hormones and toxins. It also contributes to osteoporosis because it acts as a diuretic, leaching out valuable minerals such as calcium. During menopause, women often become more sensitive to the effects of alcohol and it can exacerbate hot flashes and insomnia.
- **Try to minimize stress** by improving your diet to reduce stress on your body, as well as reducing worry in other areas of your life by embracing mental wellness exercises (see Chapter 3) or exercising more to release endorphins (see Chapter 5). The arrival of menopause into an already stressful life can cause additional stress with changing hormones; and long-term stress can suppress your immune system and affect your digestion, liver, heart health, and bones.

HOW TO USE THIS CHAPTER

This chapter shows you how to maximize your diet for optimum health during perimenopause, menopause, and beyond. It covers the main food groups, minerals, and vitamins; good sources of each; and how you can boost your intake of them easily.

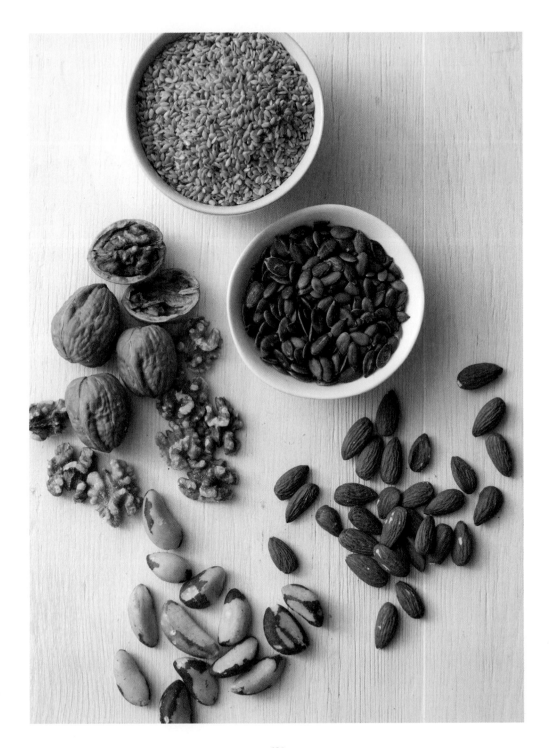

HEALTHY FATS

PROTECTS HEART | BOOSTS BRAIN | BENEFITS BONE HEALTH | PROVIDES ENERGY

Not all fats are bad. Good fats are vital for your health, especially during menopause, and include monounsaturated fats and polyunsaturated essential fatty acids such as omega-3 and omega-6 fats. These fats are needed for energy, to help absorb vitamins, and to protect your heart, brain, and bones.

Healthy fats are vital for hormonal balance and reducing inflammation as well as maintaining bone density. They can help stabilize blood sugar levels, improve insulin insensitivity, and minimize sugar cravings, which can help with weight management during menopause.

Cardiovascular disease is more prevalent in women after menopause, but a good intake of healthy fats can lower the risk of heart disease and stroke.

Current research shows a diet that includes healthy fats such as omega-3 fatty acids may be helpful in decreasing the severity of hot flashes and the frequency of night sweats. Healthy fats also contribute to preserving memory and cognitive function, and may help boost mood, which are all very important at menopause.

Healthy fats are great lubricants and can help minimize the effects of declining estrogen levels during menopause, which can cause issues such as vaginal dryness, aching joints, and thinning skin.

WHAT THEY DO

Healthy fats slow the rate at which the stomach empties, thus making carbohydrates slower releasing, boosting metabolism, and making you less insulin resistant. They also lower LDL (bad) cholesterol and increase HDL (good) cholesterol, lower blood pressure, and help prevent atherosclerosis.

GOOD SOURCES

- **Oily fish** including salmon, mackerel, herrings, sardines, swordfish, and tuna are excellent sources of healthy fats.
- **Oils such as** extra virgin olive oil, sunflower oil, sesame oil, and avocado oil.
- **Avocados, seeds, and nuts** including flaxseeds, chia seeds, and walnuts.

HOW TO BOOST YOUR INTAKE

- **Eat oily fish** at least three times a week.
- **Add avocado**, seeds, and nuts to a salad.
- **Mix flaxseeds** or chia seeds with oatmeal or yogurt and enjoy for breakfast.

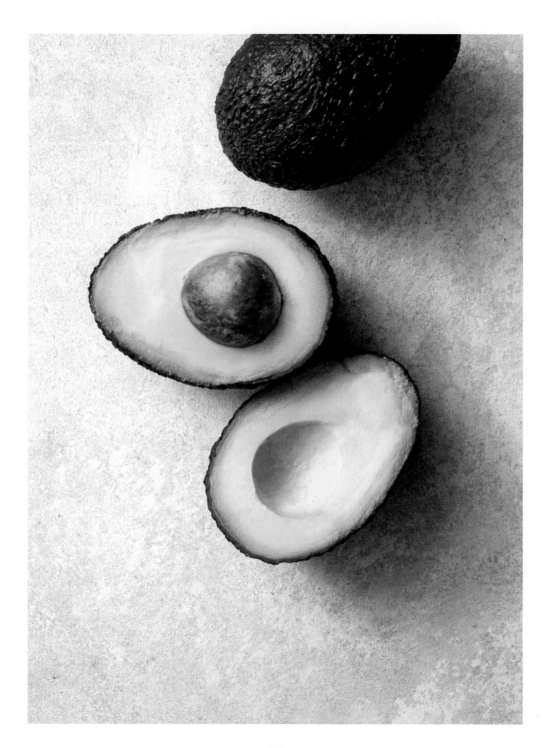

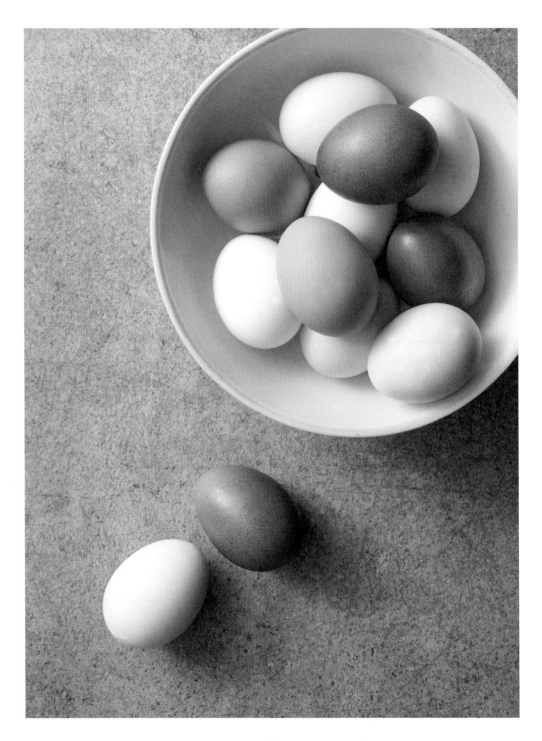

HIGH-QUALITY PROTEIN

BUILDS BONES AND MUSCLES I BALANCES BLOOD SUGAR I BENEFITS SKIN

Most processes in the body depend on protein, which is found in all body cells and is vital for good health. Ensuring you have enough high-quality protein—complete protein with all the necessary amino acids—will benefit your immune system, bones and muscles, hormone levels, skin, and hair during menopause.

Protein is essential for cell growth, tissue repair, a strong immune system, detoxification, and keeping blood sugar levels balanced. It is also crucial for maintaining and building muscles and bones, and can help negate decreasing muscle mass and bone strength, linked to declining estrogen at menopause.

Protein is needed by hormones that regulate your digestive system and thyroid. It is also important for the sex hormones. As sex hormones decline during menopause, if you do not eat enough protein and healthy fats (see page 132), your body will find it hard to make the necessary sex hormones and maintain a good hormonal balance.

WHAT IT DOES
Protein is made up of amino acids, which are the building blocks of every cell and are needed to maintain and build muscle mass and bone density, and repair tissues. Protein is also used by enzymes to help break down, digest, and absorb food.

Eating protein helps balance blood sugar levels and reduce cravings, and keeps you feeling full, all of which are important for weight management during menopause.

GOOD SOURCES
- **Chicken, turkey, meat, eggs,** fish, seafood, cottage cheese, and Greek yogurt.
- **There are many** good vegetarian sources of protein including lentils, chickpeas, whole grains, pulses, nuts, seaweed, quinoa, hemp seeds, chia seeds, tofu, and tempeh.

HOW TO BOOST YOUR INTAKE
- **Eat protein throughout the day** to keep you feeling full. Enjoy snacks such as a handful of nuts, seeded protein bars, or hard-boiled eggs.
- **Switch to Greek yogurt**, which has twice as much protein as traditional yogurt.
- **To salads add:** chicken, tuna, salmon, tofu, shrimp, walnuts, quinoa, or pumpkin seeds.
- **Make a protein shake:** blend bananas, almond butter, rolled oats, soy milk, and ice.

GOOD CARBOHYDRATES

PROVIDES ENERGY **I** BOOSTS AND BALANCES MOOD **I** AIDS WEIGHT MANAGEMENT

Carbohydrates are the body's primary source of energy in a healthy, balanced diet. Slow-release or complex carbohydrates are considered "good carbs." These are essential because they provide an even flow of glucose, which can help negate menopausal symptoms such as weight gain and fluctuations in mood.

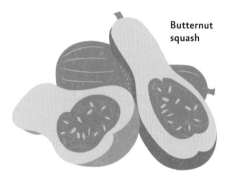

Butternut squash

Eating unrefined carbohydrates helps maintain constant energy and avoid a roller-coaster of blood sugar highs and lows. This can help you avoid or relieve many menopausal symptoms such as mood swings, cravings for sweet foods, and weight gain. Good carbs also benefit intestinal function due to their high fiber content, reducing the risk of constipation, which is a common problem during menopause.

WHAT THEY DO

Eating unrefined carbohydrates will provide a supply of slow-release energy throughout the day. Choose complex carbohydrates (such as whole grains, fruit, and vegetables), rather than simple refined carbohydrates (such as processed foods, cakes, and pastries) because simple carbohydrates are quickly digested and absorbed by the body. In contrast, complex carbohydrates take time to digest and are a stable source of energy. You can also slow the release of glucose from carbohydrates by eating it with high-quality protein (see page 135).

GOOD SOURCES

- **Whole grains such as quinoa**, brown rice, buckwheat, oats, and corn.
- **Fruit and vegetables** including butternut squash, sweet potatoes, broccoli, bananas, blueberries, apples, and citrus fruit.
- **High-fiber starchy foods** including beans and legumes.

HOW TO BOOST YOUR INTAKE

- **Choose whole grains** over refined grains.
- **Eat more legumes** such as beans, peas, and lentils. Add to stews, soups, and burgers.

WATER

REHYDRATES I BOOSTS MOOD I ALLEVIATES CONSTIPATION I SOOTHES HEADACHES

Staying hydrated is vital for your overall health at any time of life, but is especially important around perimenopause and menopause because it may feel as if your body is "drying out" due to declining estrogen levels. Drinking enough water can help improve your skin, mood, digestion, and energy levels.

Dehydration occurs when you do not drink enough water and can cause mood swings, dry skin, muscle cramps, headaches, food cravings, constipation, bladder problems, memory issues, and fatigue. Simply drinking enough—about eight glasses of water each day—can help to relieve these symptoms.

During menopause, women often experience dry skin due to declining estrogen levels, but by drinking enough water, skin will appear plumper, stiffness and discomfort in joints can ease, and hot flashes and night sweats are likely to improve because water also helps with body temperature regulation.

WHAT IT DOES

Water is vital for life and has many functions, being used for digestion, transportation and absorption of nutrients, circulation, and flushing away of waste products. It is also essential for the creation of saliva and the lubrication of joints, and acts as a shock absorber for the brain.

GOOD SOURCES
- **Bottled water is good,** or try coconut water.
- **Enjoy herbal teas** such as nettle or fennel.
- **Eat water-rich foods** such as watermelon, strawberries, peaches, oranges, and broths.

HOW TO BOOST YOUR INTAKE
- **Have a glass of** warm water and lemon in the morning to kick-start your metabolism.
- **Keep a bottle** of water handy so you get into the habit of regularly sipping water.
- **For variety,** infuse your water with fresh herbs, fruits, and vegetables (see box, below).

FLAVORED WATER

Enjoy a hydrating and refreshing drink.
- Add slices of lemon and the juice of half a lemon to a glass of plain water. Add cucumber and mint, leave to infuse, then serve cold.

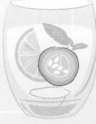

Citrus and mint water

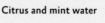

FIBER

BENEFITS DIGESTION I AIDS WEIGHT MANAGEMENT I SUPPORTS COLON HEALTH

Eating enough fiber is essential to keep your digestive system healthy. Fiber is what good gut bacteria thrives on, and having enough fiber in your diet can help keep away menopausal symptoms such as constipation, flatulence, bloating, and cravings for unhealthy foods.

Fiber helps balance blood sugar levels, which prevents spikes and crashes and can reduce cravings, which are issues for many menopausal women. It can promote weight loss by making you feel fuller faster and stay full for longer. Eating fiber-rich foods helps your body get rid of waste products and reduces the risk of diseases such as Type 2 diabetes, heart disease, and colon cancer.

Declining estrogen levels during menopause can cause bad cholesterol levels to rise, but soluble fiber aids in removing bad cholesterol from the body before absorption.

WHAT IT DOES

There are two types of fiber: soluble and insoluble. Soluble fiber is broken down by the gut and helps to soften stools and increase their frequency, which can relieve constipation. It binds with cholesterol from food and helps you to excrete it.

Insoluble fiber works like a broom through the intestines, assisting in eliminating solid waste and adding bulk to the stool to stop constipation and keep bowel movements regular.

GOOD SOURCES

- **Fruit and vegetables** such as carrots, broccoli, apples, pears, and berries.
- **Lentils, chickpeas,** and beans.
- **Whole grains,** oats, barley, nuts, and seeds.

HOW TO BOOST YOUR INTAKE

- **Leave the skin on** vegetables.
- **Eat high-fiber cereals** with chia seeds.
- **Add lentils** and beans to stews or curries.

QUINOA BERRY PORRIDGE

Breakfast is the perfect time to add more fibre to your diet.

- Mix 40g (1½oz) of quinoa with 100ml (3½fl oz) of coconut milk and a pinch of cinnamon. Cook for 5–10 minutes.
- Top with raspberries, chopped almonds, pumpkin seeds, and flax seeds and serve.

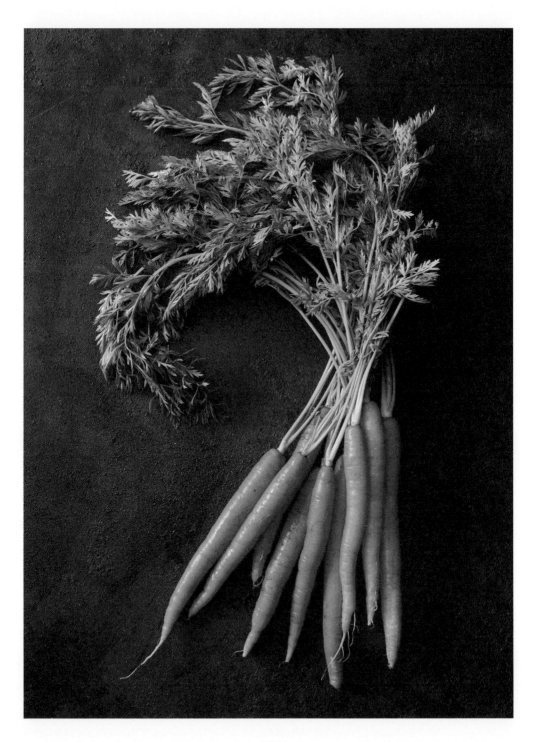

B VITAMINS

PROTECTS HEART I AIDS WEIGHT MANAGEMENT I BENEFITS DIGESTION I CALMS

For many women, stress levels can dramatically increase when going through menopause. Emotional, physical, and physiological factors all contribute to menopausal stress, but whatever the cause, B vitamins play a crucial role in managing this stress and can quickly become depleted.

B vitamins are a varied class of water-soluble vitamins including B1 (thiamine), B9 (folic acid), and B12 (cobalamin). They are involved in energy production, digestion, and fat metabolism, so ensuring you have an adequate intake can help with energy levels and weight maintenance. They are vital for managing stress, good liver function, and a healthy heart.

During menopause, women often become deficient in vitamin B12, which is required for cognitive function. This deficiency has been linked to irritability, difficulty managing stress, and insomnia.

WHAT THEY DO

B vitamins have a complex role to play in your body. They help with stress management, support estrogen production and the nervous system, and are necessary for good adrenal health.

GOOD SOURCES

- **Beef, poultry**, liver, fish, and eggs.
- **Fortified bread**, whole grains, beans, nuts, seeds, cereals, nutritional yeast, and plant-based milks are particularly good vegan and vegetarian sources of B12.
- **Vegetables,** in particular dark green leafy vegetables such as spinach and kale, plus avocados and mushrooms.

HOW TO BOOST YOUR INTAKE

- **Cook poached eggs** on tomatoes, with peppers, cilantro, and feta.
- **Make a vegetable pâté** of sunflower seeds, carrots, smoked paprika, garlic salt, onion powder, fresh cilantro, and parsley.
- **Take a supplement** (see page 150).

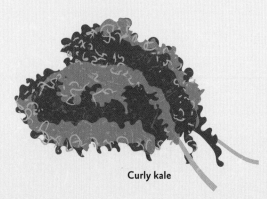

Curly kale

VITAMIN D

BENEFITS BONE AND MUSCLE HEALTH I BOOSTS MOOD I AIDS IMMUNITY

Vitamin D is produced mostly in the skin in response to sunlight, which converts it into its active form, but it can also be obtained from food and supplements. It plays a central role in many body processes and is particularly crucial during menopause because it can help improve mood and maintain bone density.

Vitamin D helps you absorb the right amount of calcium, which is vital for strong and healthy bones, particularly as you approach menopause when bone density is declining. It is also essential for maintaining muscle mass and a healthy immune system.

Many people, especially those who live in sun-deprived climates or spend little time outdoors, are deficient in vitamin D. One of the reasons why some people feel low in the winter could be a lack of vitamin D, so boosting levels may also improve mood.

HOW TO GET VITAMIN D

- Most people can make enough vitamin D in the summer months when out in the sun daily for short periods. If out for longer periods, always cover up or wear sunscreen to avoid burning.
- Take a supplement in the winter months (see page 150).
- About 10 percent of vitamin D intake is from food, so choose food rich in it.

WHAT IT DOES

Vitamin D functions more like a hormone than a vitamin. It helps with the absorption of calcium, and a lack of vitamin D can upset the all-around hormone balance.

GOOD SOURCES

- **Oily fish** such as sardines, herrings, mackerel, and salmon.
- **Free-range** and organic eggs.
- **Mushrooms** including morel, shiitake, and chanterelle, grown outdoors with natural sunlight or indoors with UV light.
- **Foods fortified with vitamin D** such as dairy products, cereals, and orange juice.

HOW TO BOOST YOUR INTAKE

- **Enjoy sardines** and avocado on toast.
- **Stir-fry** mushrooms and add to salads or pasta.

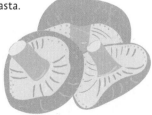

Shiitake mushrooms

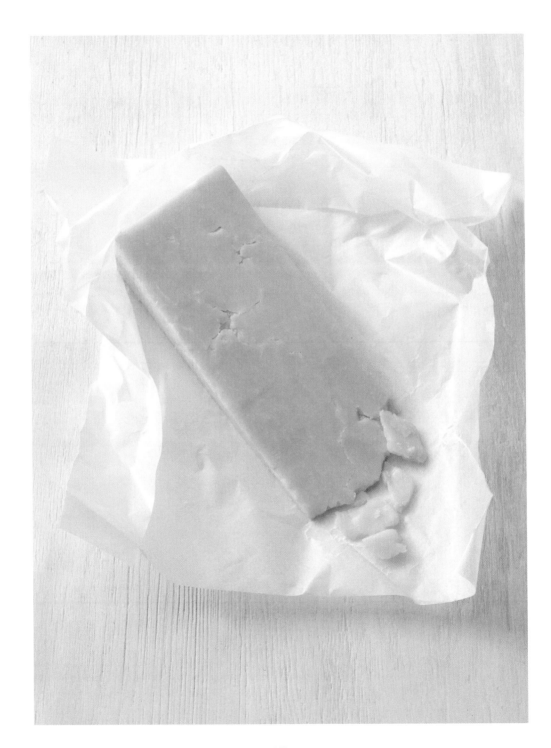

CALCIUM

BUILDS BONES AND MUSCLE I BOOSTS MOOD I PROTECTS HEART

Postmenopausal women account for 80 percent of all cases of osteoporosis because estrogen production declines rapidly at menopause. Women can lose up to 20 percent of their bone density in the five to seven years after menopause, but getting enough calcium can help maintain bone health.

When your body doesn't have sufficient calcium to perform its functions, it is taken from your bones. If this is ongoing, you can end up with osteopenia or osteoporosis, which increases the risk of bone fractures. By ensuring you have enough calcium in your diet you can help protect your bones during menopause.

Having low levels of calcium can also contribute to anxiety, stress, mood swings, depression, and sleep disturbances, which are troubling symptoms seen at menopause. Boosting your intake can therefore help with your mood and stress levels.

WHAT IT DOES

Calcium is needed for building and maintaining healthy bones; it enables your blood to clot, your muscles to contract, and your heart to beat. It is necessary for maintaining healthy communication between the brain and other parts of the body, as well as playing a role in muscle and cardiovascular function.

GOOD SOURCES

- **Dairy products** such as milk and cheese.
- **Green leafy vegetables** including broccoli, spinach, kale, cabbage, and bok choi.
- **Soy products** including tofu and tempeh.
- **Beans, lentils,** nuts, seeds, and dried fruit.
- **Sardines** and canned salmon.

HOW TO BOOST YOUR INTAKE

- **Snack on a small handful** of calcium-rich nuts such as Brazil nuts or almonds.
- **Enjoy a variety of** green leafy vegetables.
- **Take a supplement** (see page 151).

GREEN SMOOTHIE

Green smoothies are naturally good sources of calcium, as well as being loaded with vitamins and minerals.

- Blend a combination of two or three of the following calcium-rich foods: green leafy vegetables such as kale or spinach, oranges, figs, celery, almond or soy milk, and pure coconut water.

MAGNESIUM

AIDS MUSCLE AND NERVE FUNCTION **I** BOOSTS MOOD **I** IMPROVES SLEEP **I** CALMS

Magnesium is vital for health and well-being and is found in every cell in the body. However, it is one of the most common nutritional deficiencies in menopausal women. Without sufficient magnesium, fatigue, sleep problems, low mood, and muscle aches can appear or get worse during midlife.

Magnesium helps to ensure good nerve, muscle, and heart function. It regulates blood pressure, blood glucose, and energy levels, all of which can be affected by dwindling estrogen at menopause.

Magnesium helps relieve stress because it dampens down the production of cortisol, the body's main stress hormone. Magnesium is quickly depleted during times of stress, so more is needed. Adding magnesium-rich foods to your diet can therefore improve your anxiety and stress levels, as well as your sleep, which is particularly important for menopausal women, who often have disturbed sleep.

WHAT IT DOES
Magnesium is involved in more than 300 biochemical reactions in the body, and all organs need magnesium to function properly. It helps maintain proper levels of important nutrients such as potassium, zinc, and calcium (see page 143), which is needed for bone strength and density.

It also activates vitamin D (see page 141), which is important for calcium regulation and maintaining bone health.

A deficiency in magnesium can result in numbness, muscle cramps, and insomnia.

GOOD SOURCES
- **Fruit and vegetables** including bananas, squash, avocados, and dark green leafy vegetables such as kale and spinach.
- **Brown rice**, quinoa, lentils, and beans.
- **Cashew nuts**, almonds, walnuts, pumpkin seeds, sunflower seeds, and chia seeds.
- **Dark chocolate**—make sure it is at least 70 percent cocoa solids.

HOW TO BOOST YOUR INTAKE
- **Make a salad** with salmon, leafy greens, and pumpkin seeds.
- **Combine nuts**, seeds, and raw cacao to make protein balls.
- **Blend bananas**, strawberries, spinach, and almond milk to make a smoothie.
- **Take a supplement** (see page 151).

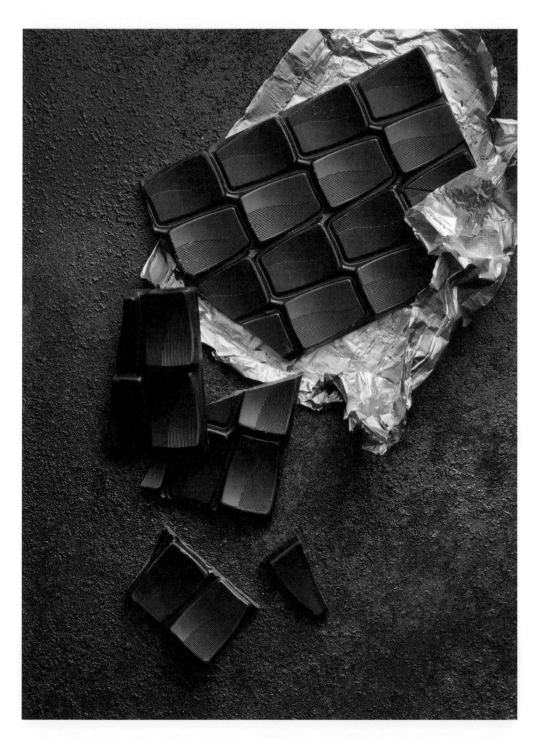

PREBIOTICS AND PROBIOTICS

BENEFITS DIGESTION I AIDS IMMUNITY I BOOSTS AND BALANCES MOOD

Prebiotics promote the growth of beneficial microorganisms in the gut. Probiotics are microbes considered to be nature's antibodies. Both are essential for a healthy gut, which is vital for overall health and immunity and can help with common menopausal symptoms such as mood swings and digestive issues.

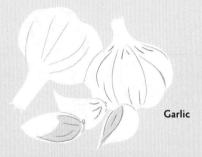

Garlic

Prebiotics are nondigestible fibrous foods that have many benefits, from improving blood sugar control and appetite regulation to supporting bone and skin health; all of which can be troublesome during menopause.

Probiotics are live bacteria and yeasts (found in fermented foods) that have a beneficial effect on the immune system, digestive health, sleep, metabolism, and recycling of hormones. They can help with menopausal bloating and moodiness.

Abdominal weight gain can be a problem for many menopausal women, but research is increasingly linking the diversity and composition of gut bacteria to weight, and showing how friendly bacteria may help with weight loss.

WHAT THEY DO

Prebiotics feed the good bacteria in the gut, while probiotics increase the number of good bacteria in the gut.

GOOD SOURCES

- **Prebiotics:** garlic, onions, leeks, asparagus, apricots, artichokes, chickpeas, beets, prunes, and Brussels sprouts.
- **Probiotics:** live yogurt, sauerkraut, tempeh, kombucha, miso, kimchi, kefir, live apple cider vinegar, and pickles.

HOW TO BOOST YOUR INTAKE

- **Enjoy natural organic** yogurt with fruit.
- **Add sauerkraut** to salads or burgers, or blend with cream cheese to make a tasty dip.
- **Take a supplement** (see page 151).

DETOXIFYING FOODS

REGULATES HORMONES I AIDS WEIGHT MANAGEMENT I BENEFITS DIGESTION

The liver, stomach, kidneys, adrenal glands, and lymphatic systems work to keep the body free of toxins and at optimal health. Toxicity can be especially problematic for women experiencing hormonal changes during menopause, so it's important to eat foods that can help to detoxify and improve health.

A healthy liver is essential for detoxification and also for weight loss. If the liver is overburdened it will force other detoxifying organs such as the skin and lymph nodes to work overtime, resulting in hormone imbalances, bloating, and poor health.

WHAT THEY DO
Detoxifying foods help ensure that the liver, the body's primary detox organ, is functioning at optimal levels. It is crucial that the liver can work effectively as it performs over 500 functions: it produces amino acids and enzymes to metabolize fat, protein, and carbohydrates and helps regulate blood sugar levels. It also helps synthesize hormones and store vitamins.

GOOD SOURCES
- **Water** (see page 137).
- **Fruit** such as lemons, berries, papaya, and pineapple.
- **Vegetables** such as cabbage, broccoli, cauliflower, kale, beets, and radishes.

- **Fermented foods** including kefir, live yogurt, sauerkraut, and kimchi.
- **Herbs and spices** including parsley, ginger, rosemary, lemongrass, and peppermint.

HOW TO BOOST YOUR INTAKE
- **Drink smoothies** made with fresh fruit and vegetables.
- **Make a detox salad** of beets, carrots, walnuts, and parsley with an olive oil, lemon juice, and apple cider vinegar dressing.
- **Drink herbal teas**—try chamomile, lemon, dandelion, red clover, nettle, or green tea.

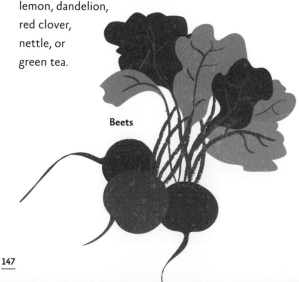

Beets

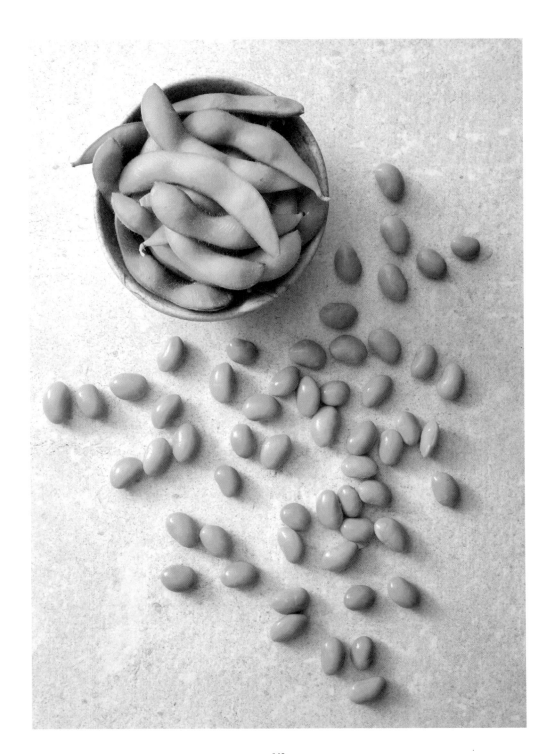

PHYTOESTROGENS

REDUCES HOT FLASHES I BOOSTS MOOD I REGULATES HORMONES

Phytoestrogens (plant estrogens) are naturally occurring compounds found in a wide range of plant foods, most notably soy. Research has shown that women in countries such as Japan, who eat a diet rich in soy, have fewer menopausal symptoms, in particular hot flashes, than women in Western cultures.

Plant foods containing phytoestrogens are hormone-balancing and have the added nutritional benefits of providing protein, fiber, vitamins, and minerals. Research indicates that a regular intake of phytoestrogens may help manage or alleviate menopausal symptoms such as hot flashes and night sweats, combat dips in mood and energy, improve cognitive function and memory, and protect against heart disease. Phytoestrogens may also help lower the risk of osteoporosis and breast cancer.

WHAT THEY DO

Phytoestrogens are part of a group of chemicals called isoflavones. They imitate estrogen because their chemical structure is similar to—but weaker than—estrogen in the body. They occupy estrogen receptors and somehow alter the action of these receptors, stimulating them in some areas of the body while blocking them in other areas. See also page 40.

GOOD SOURCES

Soy products and flaxseeds have the highest levels—soy products contain isoflavones; flaxseeds contain lignans.

- **Soy products** such as tofu, soy milk, tempeh, soybeans, and edamame beans.
- **Nuts and seeds** including flaxseeds, sesame seeds, sunflower seeds, walnuts, and almonds.
- **Legumes** such as lentils, chickpeas, mung beans, aduki beans, and kidney beans.
- **Fruit and vegetables,** in particular yams, green leafy vegetables, and berries.

HOW TO BOOST YOUR INTAKE

- **Add tofu to** scrambled eggs, smoothies, stir-fries, soups, or salads. Use it alongside or in place of meat.
- **Make a seed mix** by combining two parts flaxseeds, one part sunflower seeds, and one part sesame seeds. Add to smoothies or sprinkle on porridge, yogurt, or salads.
- **Enhance a Bolognese sauce** by adding lentils, chickpeas, spinach, or tofu.

SUPPLEMENTS

Supplements can be an important addition to your diet during menopause to address deficiencies in key vitamins and minerals, as well as boosting your physical and mental well-being and overall health. However, supplements are not a substitute for a healthy diet, and eating a range of nutritious foods is vital.

Menopause can cause a lot of stress on your body and this can often lead to vitamin and mineral deficiencies. Supplements can provide extra support to help you go through this phase of life smoothly.

The supplements listed here can help improve hormonal, bone, brain, and gut health during menopause. Increasing your intake of nutrients such as calcium, zinc, vitamin D, magnesium, omega-3 fats, and vitamin E can make a big difference to the bone and heart health. See also page 219.

Check with your physician before taking supplements, and tell them what you are taking before surgery or procedures. Look for supplements that have USP verification.

VITAMIN SUPPLEMENTS

B VITAMINS

B vitamins are helpful during times of stress. They work in harmony together, so a deficiency in one can affect the efficiency of others. Aim for a good intake of all the B vitamins. See also page 140.

VITAMIN C

Vitamin C is an important antioxidant and powerful immune system booster. It helps build up collagen, which gives skin and tissues elasticity, and is essential for strong and healthy bones.

VITAMIN D

Vitamin D supports the immune system and is essential for bone health. It is mainly obtained via sunlight, so it is advisable to take a supplement during the winter when sun is scarce. See also page 141.

VITAMIN E

Vitamin E helps improve immune function and control inflammation, and may ease stress on the body. Choose a complete family of compounds and ideally take with vitamin C and Co-Q10.

MINERAL SUPPLEMENTS

CALCIUM

Calcium is essential for good bone health, helping prevent the natural decline in bone density that can lead to osteoporosis. Calcium may also improve blood sugar balance. Take with vitamin D for increased bone strength; but be careful not to take too much. See also page 143.

MAGNESIUM

Magnesium is vital for bone health, heart health, and blood pressure. It converts vitamin D into its active form, which enables calcium to be absorbed. It has a calming effect, easing menopausal symptoms such as irritability and anxiety, as well as helping with insomnia. See also page 144.

ZINC

Zinc is essential for many regulatory systems in the body, including the healthy production of the thyroid hormones. It also plays a part in appetite control, so it may help with weight maintenance. Zinc works with vitamin D to help boost calcium absorption and preserve bone density.

OTHER SUPPLEMENTS

ISOFLAVONES

There is some evidence that phytoestrogens/ isoflavones taken as a supplement can help with menopausal symptoms such as hot flashes. However, check with your health-care provider before taking, especially if you have had a hormone-responsive disease. See also page 149.

OMEGA-3 FATS

Omega-3 fats have many beneficial anti-inflammatory effects on the heart, brain, bones, and joints. They help keep skin and hair soft and supple, may boost cognition, and can help reduce menopausal symptoms such as hot flashes and mood swings. See also page 132.

PROBIOTICS

Probiotics can help correct the imbalance of bacteria in the gut. Poor digestion due to hormone imbalances affects the balance of bacteria in the gut, but probiotics can help maintain a healthy gut, which in turn benefits hormonal health and general well-being. See also page 146.

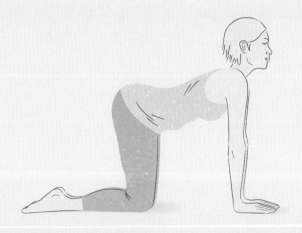

EXERCISE

INTRODUCTION

Exercise is one of the most powerful tools you have in your toolbox to alleviate and in some cases reverse the most serious physiological impacts of menopause. All types of exercise will bring you health benefits, but some forms of exercise are particularly advantageous during menopause.

BENEFITS OF EXERCISE

You probably know that exercise is good for you, but may have lost sight of just how good it is. Through regular exercise you can slow down and even reverse the loss of muscle mass and bone density; decrease your risk of osteoporosis and cardiovascular disease; and lose weight, including stubborn belly fat. Exercise can also improve your mood and boost mental health, while giving you a chance to enjoy the outdoors and socialize.

MUSCLE AND BONE HEALTH

Both men and women gradually lose muscle mass and bone density with age. For women, estrogen levels start to fluctuate and become unpredictable during perimenopause and then drop to a low level at menopause, which often accelerates the deterioration of bone health and muscle size and strength. This can lead to osteoporosis and sarcopenia (loss of muscle), resulting in old-age immobility and frailty. Though these are a natural part of the aging process, it is now known that adequate exercise combined with good nutrition (particularly eating sufficient high-quality protein—see page 135) can not only stop the natural decline, but often reverse it. In this sense, exercise can help you stay young.

HEART HEALTH

Cardiovascular disease is the number-one cause of death for women in the US—1 in 5 will die from it. High blood pressure and hardening of the arteries (sometimes exacerbated by being overweight) conspire to cause strokes, heart attacks, and coronary heart disease. Estrogen has a protective effect that is reduced as levels decline in menopause, resulting in a heightened risk of heart disease. Adequate exercise, particularly when combined with maintaining a healthy weight, can improve your blood pressure and other risk factors for heart disease.

MAINTAINING A HEALTHY WEIGHT

Menopause is commonly associated with weight gain, particularly an increase in fat in

" "

It is never too late to start exercising, or to try out new types of exercise. Whether it's yoga, swimming, Pilates, running, cycling, or strength training, why not give it a try and see what a difference regular exercise can make to your body, mood, and overall well-being.

the midsection of your body. If unchecked, weight gain can lead to obesity. The health consequences of obesity are well known— a substantially increased risk of heart disease and many cancers. If you are overweight, losing weight is an important step in avoiding disease and living longer.

The rate at which we lose weight may vary from person to person due to different metabolisms, genetics, and other factors, but all of us will lose weight if the calories we burn exceed the calories we consume. People often overestimate the number of calories they burn from exercise and underestimate the number of calories they burn from everyday movement and activities. If you want to increase the calories you burn, the best way of doing that is simply to move more. Walk instead of driving. Take the stairs instead of the elevator.

While exercise does burn calories, it typically represents 10 percent or less of daily calorie expenditure for the average person. By all means, exercise more

to burn more calories, but also make sure your diet is on point (see also Chapter 4). If you lose weight without exercising, you will lose both fat and muscle. Menopause is a time of life when you need to try to preserve muscle mass. The only way to lose fat without losing muscle is to combine strength training with eating a good amount of high-quality protein as part of a well-balanced diet.

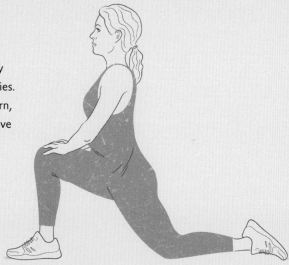

MENTAL HEALTH

Many women report heightened anxiety, low mood, and a loss of self-confidence during menopause. There is strong evidence that exercise makes you feel better and contributes positively to mental health and happiness. It's well known that exercise promotes the release of neurotransmitters in your body, such as serotonin and endorphins, which make you feel good and improve your mood. Beyond that, there is a correlation between regular exercise and reduced anxiety and depression, and increased self-confidence, although the scientific reasons are not yet fully understood.

Many forms of yoga (see pages 186–197) are relaxing and are often combined with meditation or introspection, thus having an overall calming, de-stressing effect.

HOT FLASHES AND NIGHT SWEATS

What about the so-called vasomotor symptoms of menopause—hot flashes and night sweats? Some women report that exercise seems to alleviate their symptoms, and some scientific research suggests a correlation between exercise and reduced symptoms. However, there is simply not enough scientific evidence to conclude definitively that exercise helps.

DIFFERENT TYPES OF EXERCISE

If you already exercise, consider the different types of exercise you do and its impact on your health and wellness. You may benefit from adding different types of exercise to your weekly routine. If you do not exercise (or not as much as you know you should), we give tips for getting started, as well as straightforward programs you can follow (see pages 162–197). Find out what suits you and vary the exercise you do.

You can get more out of your exercise regimen if you mix it up and make it fun. If you're not keen on lifting weights, try a circuit class that includes strength training. If you don't enjoy running on a treadmill, consider hill walking or spin classes, or try a new form of dance.

CARDIOVASCULAR EXERCISE

Cardiovascular exercise raises your heart rate and is the most effective exercise to improve your overall fitness levels and reduce your

Strength training is the most effective type of exercise to maintain lean muscle mass and prevent the loss of muscle strength as we age and as we experience declining estrogen levels during menopause.

BEST TYPES OF EXERCISE

FOR FLEXIBILITY

Pilates, yoga, dancing, swimming, and martial arts such as t'ai chi, judo, and karate can increase your flexibility, keeping you supple and mobile and preventing stiffness during menopause.

FOR MOOD

Yoga, or exercising with friends, for example, jogging or doing a dance class together, can boost mood. Also try team sports such as netball or football—it's even better if the sport is played outside.

FOR STRENGTH

Weightlifting, training using your bodyweight or resistance bands, and circuit classes are excellent ways to build bones and muscles, helping to maintain strength during menopause.

FOR THE HEART

Jogging, running, cycling, hill walking, kayaking, dancing, circuit classes, boxing, tennis, squash, swimming, and using a treadmill or rowing machine are all good forms of cardiovascular exercise.

risk of heart disease, which increases during menopause due to the decline of protective estrogen (see page 154). See box (above) for good examples of cardiovascular exercise that you can do either outdoors or indoors.

Some cardiovascular exercise is high impact, driving force through your joints, such as jumping or running and sports that require them. Although it's a great form of exercise, be mindful that high-impact exercise can put you at greater risk of injury, especially as bone density declines during and after menopause. Other cardiovascular exercise is low-impact, driving little or no force through your joints, such as swimming.

MOBILITY AND FLEXIBILITY EXERCISES

Mobility and flexibility are about the ability of your muscles to contract and extend and the ability of your joints to accommodate a full range of motion. As we age, our mobility and flexibility naturally decline, and this is often exacerbated by joint pain, which is a common symptom of menopause. While all movement can improve mobility, exercises that include static and dynamic stretching will help (see box, above).

STRENGTH TRAINING

Strength training is the best exercise to redress some of the most profound

TIPS TO STAY MOTIVATED

LOVE THE SPORT

Start by doing something you know you enjoy, such as yoga, dancing, swimming, tennis, or hiking outdoors.

TUNE IN

Listen to your favorite music or a good podcast to keep your mind off the passage of time while you are exercising.

MAKE IT SOCIAL

Exercise with a friend or join an exercise class where you will meet like-minded women. Socializing makes exercise more fun.

BOOK IT UP

Join a gym, rec center, or fitness studio, or hire a fitness professional. If you put it on your calendar, you are more likely to do it.

TALK ABOUT IT

Tell your colleagues and family about your exercise plans so they can give you the space in your day and the support that you need.

SEE PROGRESS

Monitor your progress. Take photos to show how your body is changing. Seeing a difference can be a very powerful motivator.

physiological impacts of menopause—delaying, preventing, or even reversing the loss of bone density and muscle mass.

Strength training works specific muscles by imposing resistance on muscular contraction in order to strengthen them and to improve their endurance. Lifting weights is the most common example, but strength training also includes bodyweight exercises (see page 162) and using simple kit such as resistance bands (see page 170) or a TRX.

CHANGING PERCEPTIONS

An increasing number of women at midlife are recognizing the importance of strength training to their health through perimenopause, menopause, and beyond. In the past some women were put off by the thought of a commercial gym environment, but gyms can be warm, friendly, supportive places where a novice is embraced, assisted, and encouraged. There are also many alternatives to commercial gyms, such as recreation centers, small fitness studios, or working with a personal trainer. You can also enjoy strength training in your own home, doing bodyweight workouts without equipment (see page 162), or using equipment such as resistance bands (see page 170).

A common misconception is that lifting weights will give you bulky muscles. Nothing could be further from the truth. Women naturally produce only a fraction of muscle-promoting hormones that men do, so will only preserve or modestly enhance muscle mass and strength when strength training.

HOW MUCH EXERCISE IS ENOUGH?

Though recommendations vary, most government guidelines in the developed world recommend a minimum of 2.5 to 5 hours per week of moderate exercise or 1.5 to 2.5 hours per week of vigorous exercise to gain health benefits. More is better, but only to a point. The most important objective is to get started and make exercise a sustainable habit, ingrained in your lifestyle. It's better to start small than not at all.

GETTING STARTED

If you are new to exercise, the first thing to know is that menopause is not an impediment, but a great reason to get started. If you have had a recent injury or surgery, or if you are ill or have certain health conditions, such as high blood pressure, heart disease, arthritis, or diabetes, consult your doctor before getting started. If you are clear to go, there are many forms of exercise you can start on your own, such as brisk walking or cycling. You can join a class run by a qualified exercise professional and do yoga, dance, CrossFit, or interval training.

Many people struggle to get started, or have tried in the past and not yet succeeded. Establishing new habits and making them a permanent, sustainable part of your lifestyle can be challenging. Finding your personal motivation to exercise is often the key to your success. A nagging partner is weak motivation and will rarely sustain new behaviors. Make yourself the center of your motivation. "I want to be fit and healthy so I can enjoy sports/I can play with my grandchildren." The ultimate goal, of course, is to make exercise part of your life: "I exercise because that is what I do to lead a healthy and happy life."

If you do exercise regularly but find that you are stuck in a rut or following an exercise regimen that is no longer working for you, you may find that adapting your routine and incorporating new types of exercise will put you in a stronger position to navigate the menopause transition.

SAFETY FIRST

If you are new to a form of exercise, such as strength training, you need to ensure that your technique and body positioning are correct and safe in order to minimize any risk of injury. The best way to do that is to join a class led by a qualified fitness professional or hire an experienced personal trainer, at least to get you started.

In time, almost everyone who exercises regularly enjoys doing so. You may also find that having an exercise regimen will help you feel more in control of your life, helping your mental well-being.

Start by taking small steps. If you would like to try running, but are new to it, start by walking for two minutes, then jogging for 30 seconds, then repeat for a total of 15 minutes. Every few days increase the amount of time you spend jogging. Within a few weeks, you are likely to be a regular runner who looks forward to the next run. You can apply the same gradual approach to any new type of exercise you decide to do.

THE EXERCISE PROGRAMS

The three strength training workouts featured here have been designed for maximum health benefits at menopause. They focus on building strength to maintain healthy bones and muscles and can be started well before menopause, or during perimenopause or menopause.

The workouts include a simple bodyweight program you don't need any equipment for (see page 162); a workout using resistance bands (see page 170); and a gym-based workout using weights (see page 178).

For the yoga sequence (see page 186), we present a mixed Yang and Yin program. This promotes flexibility while calming and balancing the mind and body.

The programs can serve as a starting point for your exercise journey, or complement your current exercise regimen. Although you may want to prioritize one type of exercise in order to reach your personal goals or address your personal concerns, there is value in including different forms of exercise in your routine.

Ideally, do your chosen strength training workout and the yoga sequence a couple of times a week each, combined with days doing other exercise you enjoy, and allowing for rest days.

WARM-UP

It is important to warm up before exercising as an effective warm-up transitions you from a sedentary state to one primed for exercise (see right). It mobilizes the joints, ligaments, and surrounding muscles; activates the key muscles; and allows you to move as freely as possible while minimizing your risk of injury.

TERMINOLOGY

Rep = one complete movement of an exercise.
Rest = time spent resting after a set.
Set = a completed group of consecutive repetitions or time spent on an exercise.
Super-sets = alternating two exercises to increase the efficiency of the workout.
Tempo = time spent performing each rep through its different stages.

WARM-UP EXERCISES

These exercises are designed to be carried out before doing the workouts on pages 162–185. They cover the areas of the body where most people experience some restricted movement: the ankles, hips, spine, and shoulders.

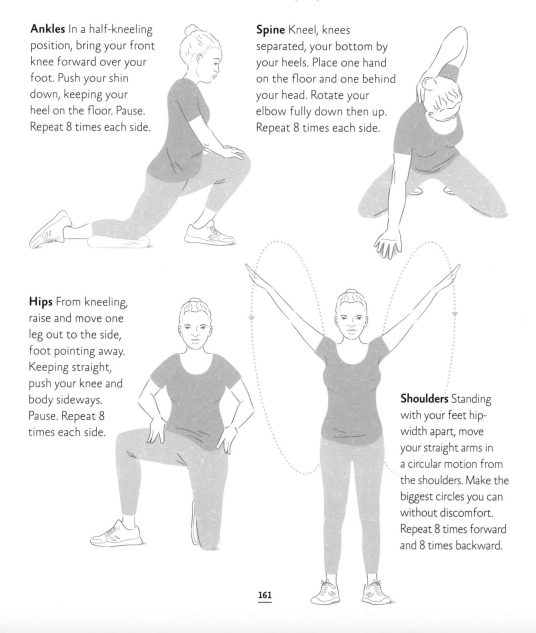

Ankles In a half-kneeling position, bring your front knee forward over your foot. Push your shin down, keeping your heel on the floor. Pause. Repeat 8 times each side.

Spine Kneel, knees separated, your bottom by your heels. Place one hand on the floor and one behind your head. Rotate your elbow fully down then up. Repeat 8 times each side.

Hips From kneeling, raise and move one leg out to the side, foot pointing away. Keeping straight, push your knee and body sideways. Pause. Repeat 8 times each side.

Shoulders Standing with your feet hip-width apart, move your straight arms in a circular motion from the shoulders. Make the biggest circles you can without discomfort. Repeat 8 times forward and 8 times backward.

BODYWEIGHT WORKOUT

This workout is low-impact, technically simple, and time-efficient, so it is ideal to do during menopause, especially if you are new to this kind of exercise. It trains all the main muscle groups with equal attention, making it balanced and comprehensive. Because it's a bodyweight-only workout, it requires no equipment and you can perform it anywhere—at home or in a park.

WHAT YOU NEED

All you need is sufficient space to perform the exercises, although you may want to use a yoga mat for the floor exercises and have pillows for the exercises where you need to kneel.

HOW TO FOLLOW THE WORKOUT

For best results, perform this workout—which takes around 45 minutes including the warm-up—at least twice a week, three times maximum, with at least one day's rest between sessions.

Some exercises have more than one version or a suggested progression—start with the easier version until you're confident.

- **Do 12–15 x Bodyweight Squats.** Rest for 30 seconds, and then do 15–45 seconds x Plank From Knees or Plank From Toes. Rest for 45–60 seconds. Repeat for 2–3 super-sets.
- **Do 8–10 x Hands Elevated Push-ups.** Rest for 30 seconds, and then do 12–15 x Glute Bridges. Rest for 45–60 seconds. Repeat for 2–3 super-sets.
- **Do 8–10 x Supported Split Squat or Reverse Lunge** for each leg. Rest for 30 seconds, and then do 10–15 x Prone Cobra. Rest for 45–60 seconds. Repeat for 2–3 super-sets.

SAFETY NOTE

To minimize your risk of injury, start with the warm-up (see page 161). If any of the exercises causes you pain, stop right away.

BODYWEIGHT SQUAT

The squat is one of the most important exercises for maintaining lower-body strength. During menopause, muscle strength naturally declines, but consistently performing squats will help build your thigh muscles in particular, assisting with everyday activities and general movement.

Reps: 12–15

Tempo: 3 seconds down, 1 second pause, 1 second up

Progression: Extend the pause in the squat position

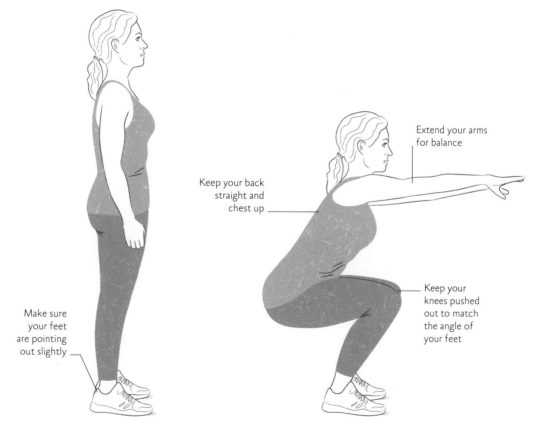

Keep your back straight and chest up

Extend your arms for balance

Make sure your feet are pointing out slightly

Keep your knees pushed out to match the angle of your feet

1 **Stand up straight** with your feet shoulder-width apart. Turn your feet out to roughly 10 and 2 o'clock. Keep your chest up to maintain a straight spine and prevent your lower back from rounding.

2 **Sit back by bending** your knees and hips at the same time. Keep your knees pushed out over your toes. Descend as low as you can without your back rounding. Hold, then push through your mid-foot to stand.

PLANK

When done correctly, the Plank is an excellent core exercise to do during menopause and beyond because it strengthens your abdominal muscles, the internal muscles surrounding your lower back, and your glutes. These core muscles help keep you balanced and stable and your spine safe.

Reps: 2–3
Hold time: 15–45 seconds
Progression: Plank from toes

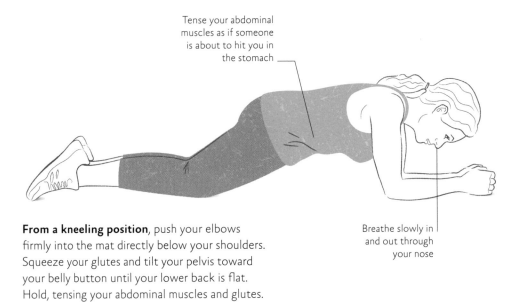

Tense your abdominal muscles as if someone is about to hit you in the stomach

Breathe slowly in and out through your nose

From a kneeling position, push your elbows firmly into the mat directly below your shoulders. Squeeze your glutes and tilt your pelvis toward your belly button until your lower back is flat. Hold, tensing your abdominal muscles and glutes.

PLANK FROM TOES

This plank variation is more challenging as it requires your core to support more of your body weight than when done from the knees. Follow the instructions above, but rest on your toes, not your knees.

Keep your knees locked by tensing your thighs

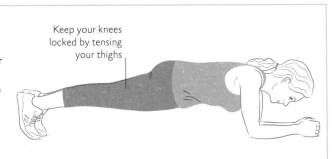

HANDS ELEVATED PUSH-UP

This push-up is essentially a Plank (see opposite) with the addition of an upper-body strength pushing movement. It works the pectorals, front of shoulders, and triceps and can help you maintain lean muscle mass and strength in your upper body, which can weaken during menopause.

Reps: 8–10
Tempo: 2 seconds down, 1-second pause, 1 second up, 1-second pause

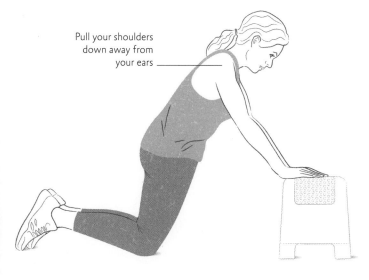

Pull your shoulders down away from your ears

1 **Kneel on the ground** and place your hands just outside shoulder-width apart on a secure raised surface. Create a plank position through your torso by keeping your glutes and abdominal muscles tight and your shoulder blades fully separated.

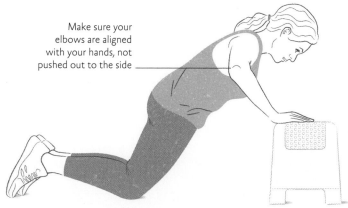

Make sure your elbows are aligned with your hands, not pushed out to the side

2 **Bend your arms** and lower your chest to a depth from which you are strong enough to push back to the starting point, while forming a 45–60 degree angle between your upper arms and torso. Hold, then push back up, maintaining a solid plank throughout the movement.

GLUTE BRIDGE

The Glute Bridge strengthens the back of your lower body. When performed correctly, it should primarily be felt in the glutes, not the lower back. Strong glutes will keep you mobile and athletic, helping prevent lower-back issues as they support the spine, which can be affected by menopause.

Reps: 12–15

Tempo: 1 second up, 1-second pause, 1 second down

Progression: Increase the pause time to 2–3 seconds

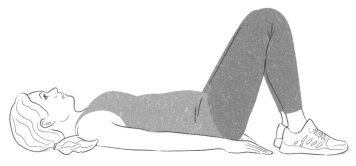

1 **Lie on your back** and bend your knees. Place your feet flat on the floor, shoulder- to hip-width apart, with your toes forward or slightly turned out. Tighten your abdominal muscles.

Pull in your abdominal muscles to prevent your back from arching

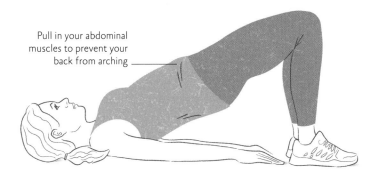

2 **Drive through your heels** to push your hips toward the ceiling until you form a straight line through your shoulders, hips, and knees. At the top, clench your glutes as tightly as possible, then slowly lower back down to the ground.

SUPPORTED SPLIT SQUAT

Split-stance leg exercises even out strength and coordination between your left and right sides, which can help to maintain your balance and mobility during menopause as your muscle performance declines. This exercise should be mastered before moving on to the Reverse Lunge (see page 168).

Reps: 8–10 per leg

Tempo: 1 second up, 1-second pause, 2 seconds down, 1-second pause

Progressions: Do without the chair. Next, the Reverse Lunge (see page 168)

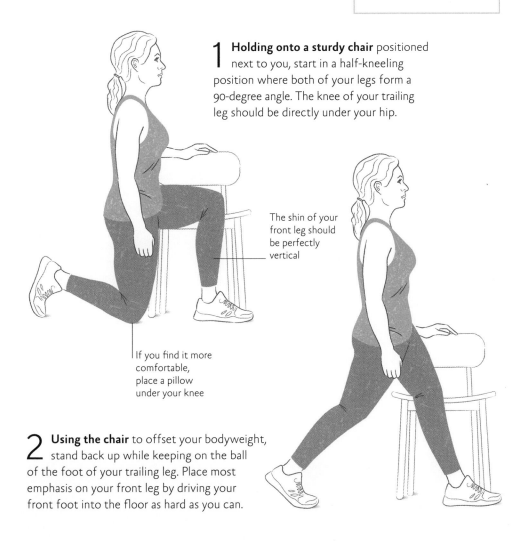

1 **Holding onto a sturdy chair** positioned next to you, start in a half-kneeling position where both of your legs form a 90-degree angle. The knee of your trailing leg should be directly under your hip.

The shin of your front leg should be perfectly vertical

If you find it more comfortable, place a pillow under your knee

2 **Using the chair** to offset your bodyweight, stand back up while keeping on the ball of the foot of your trailing leg. Place most emphasis on your front leg by driving your front foot into the floor as hard as you can.

REVERSE LUNGE

The Reverse Lunge is a dynamic split-stance leg exercise and is the safest progression from the Split Squat (see page 167). It is a very beneficial exercise to do during menopause because it can improve the strength and power of your leg muscles, as well as your general mobility.

Reps: 8–10 per leg
Tempo: 1 second back, 1 second down, 1-second pause, 1 second forward, 1-second pause

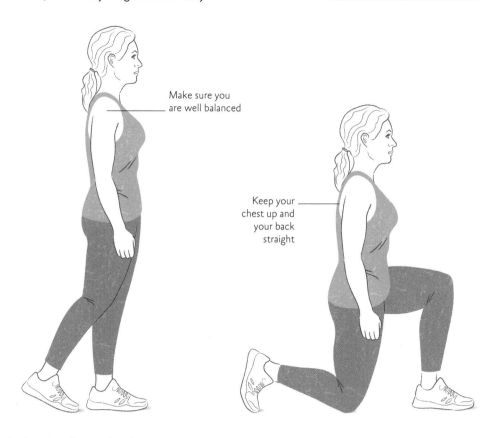

Make sure you are well balanced

Keep your chest up and your back straight

1 **Stand with your feet level**, hip-width apart, then carefully take a big stride backward as if you are stepping over a ditch. Firmly ground your leg on the ball of your foot.

2 **Lower your knee** slowly and in a controlled way until it touches the floor. Pause, then push powerfully through your front foot to "step back over the ditch without falling in" and return to the start.

PRONE COBRA

This upper-back strengthening exercise is great for improving your posture. Being stressed during menopause can mean that your shoulders become hunched up, but this key exercise pulls down the shoulders and can help you avoid or improve any shoulder issues you may have.

Reps: 10–15

Tempo: 2 seconds up, 1-second pause, 1 second down

Progression: Increase the pause time to 2–3 seconds

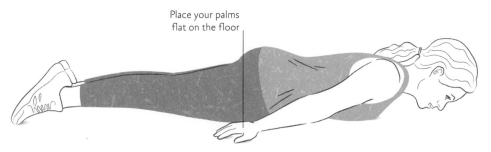

Place your palms flat on the floor

1 **Lie on the floor** on your front in an arrow shape with your palms facing down, resting on the floor. Slowly lift your chest off the floor as far as you can while keeping your feet down and your glutes as relaxed as possible.

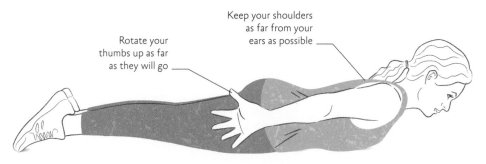

Keep your shoulders as far from your ears as possible

Rotate your thumbs up as far as they will go

2 **Keeping your shoulders down,** turn hands out to rotate thumbs toward the ceiling. Squeeze shoulder blades together, creating tension in the upper and mid-back muscle. Hold at least one second, then return to the start.

BAND WORKOUT

This simple but effective workout is an ideal way to exercise during menopause because it has all the great features of the Bodyweight Workout (see page 162), with the additional benefits of using resistance bands. Selecting the correct band gives you the ability to precisely match and develop your current strength and technique levels, helping to further strengthen key muscles.

WHAT YOU NEED

A set of resistance bands. Purchase three bands that roughly match these profiles: 5–10lbs/2–4.5kg of resistance (usually yellow), 15–25lbs/7–11kg (usually blue), and 30–60lbs/13–27kg (usually black).
    You will also need a door anchor, or a pole to attach the band to.

THE WORKOUT

For best results, perform this workout—which takes around 45 minutes including the warm-up—at least twice a week, three times maximum, with at least one day's rest between sessions.
    To progress, use a band with a higher resistance.
- **Do 12–15 x Band Goblet Squats.** Rest for 30 seconds, then do 10–12 Half-Kneeling Pallof Presses. Rest for 45–60 seconds. Repeat for 2–3 super-sets.
- **Do 10–12 x Band Floor Presses.** Rest for 30 seconds, then do 12–15 x Band Good Morning or Band Romanian Deadlifts. Rest for 45–60 seconds. Repeat for 2–3 super-sets.
- **Do 8–10 x Band Split Squats** for each leg. Rest for 30 seconds, then do 10–12 x Half-Kneeling Band Rows. Rest for 45–60 seconds. Repeat for 2–3 super-sets.

SAFETY NOTES

To minimize your risk of injury, start with the warm-up (see page 161). If any of the exercises causes you pain, stop right away.

BAND GOBLET SQUAT

In this adaptation of the Bodyweight Squat (see page 163), the increasing tension in the band as you stand provides a greater challenge to the strength of your legs. Because bone density declines during menopause, it is vital to exercise to keep your leg muscles and bones strong and healthy.

Reps: 12–15
Tempo: 3 seconds down, 1-second pause, 1 second up
Progression: Use a thicker band

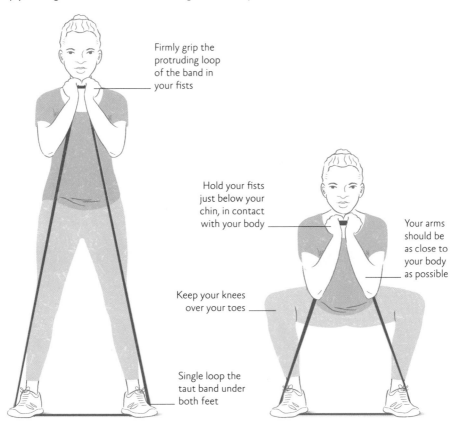

Firmly grip the protruding loop of the band in your fists

Hold your fists just below your chin, in contact with your body

Your arms should be as close to your body as possible

Keep your knees over your toes

Single loop the taut band under both feet

1 **Stand with your feet** shoulder-width apart, your feet at 10 and 2 o'clock. Place the band under your feet and grip the band loop in your fists. Press your fists together just below your chin, your elbows tucked in.

2 **Sit back by bending** your knees and hips at the same time. Keep your arms and hands locked in position. Descend as low as you can without your back rounding. Hold, then push though your mid-foot to stand.

HALF-KNEELING PALLOF PRESS

This is a great exercise to strengthen the internal core muscles that support your spine, as well as the abdominal muscles and obliques. These naturally weaken during menopause but are key for maintaining a good posture. The challenge is resisting being pulled out of position.

Reps: 10–12

Tempo: 2 seconds out, 1-second pause, 2 seconds back

Progression: Use a thicker band

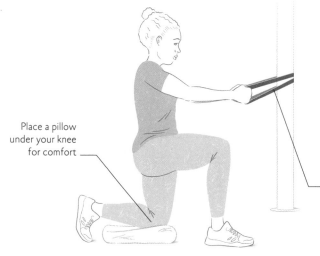

Place a pillow under your knee for comfort

1 **Anchor the band** stably to the side of you at the height of your sternum in a half-kneeling position. Grip the band in your fists and pull your hands into your sternum. Adjust the distance to create enough tension to engage your core muscles.

Double-loop the band around a pole or through a door anchor

Keep your shoulders and back straight so you don't lean forward or backward

Ensure your hands move in a perfectly straight line

Apart from your arms, your body should remain completely still

2 **Firmly ground** your front foot and trailing knee. Keeping the tension in your abdominal muscles, glutes, and legs, slowly extend your arms in a straight line. Hold, then bring your hands back to your sternum, again in a straight line.

BAND FLOOR PRESS

This is a great upper-body exercise to do during menopause because it strengthens the chest, shoulders, and triceps. By selecting an appropriate band, it is easier to match your current strength levels instead of being limited to working with your body weight.

Reps: 10–12

Tempo: 1 second up, 1-second pause, 1 second down, 1-second pause

Progression: Use a thicker band

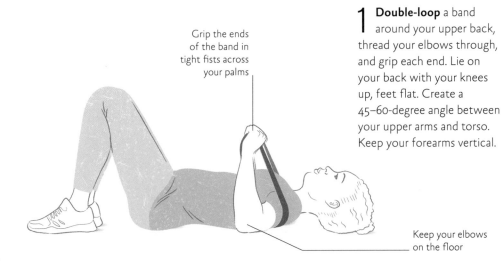

Grip the ends of the band in tight fists across your palms

1 **Double-loop** a band around your upper back, thread your elbows through, and grip each end. Lie on your back with your knees up, feet flat. Create a 45–60-degree angle between your upper arms and torso. Keep your forearms vertical.

Keep your elbows on the floor

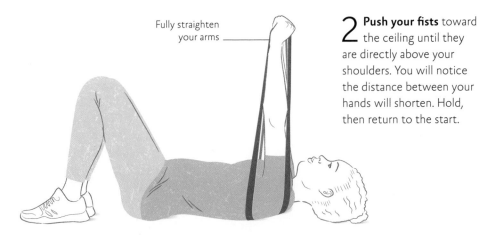

Fully straighten your arms

2 **Push your fists** toward the ceiling until they are directly above your shoulders. You will notice the distance between your hands will shorten. Hold, then return to the start.

BAND GOOD MORNING

This low-risk hip-hinge movement primarily strengthens the glutes and hamstrings, and can help improve or avoid lower-back issues that often start during menopause. The repeated movement should resemble a "bow and arrow" action as your bottom moves forward and backward.

Reps: 12–15

Tempo: 2 seconds down, 1-second pause, 1 second up, 1-second pause

Progression: Romanian Deadlift (see opposite)

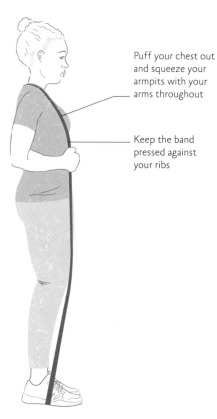

Puff your chest out and squeeze your armpits with your arms throughout

Keep the band pressed against your ribs

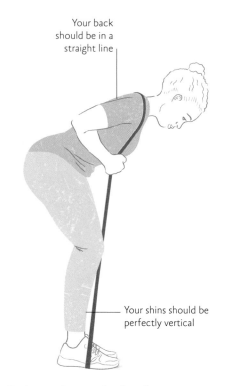

Your back should be in a straight line

Your shins should be perfectly vertical

1 **Loop a taut band** under the middle of both feet and around the back of your neck. Your feet should be hip-width apart and your toes very slightly turned out. Hold onto the band like suspenders, against your chest.

2 **Push your bottom back** as far as you can and lean forward with a straight back and bent knees—as if looking over a cliff. Hold, then push your hips forward, squeeze your glutes, and stand upright.

BAND ROMANIAN DEADLIFT

This exercise works the same muscles as the Band Good Morning (see opposite), but allows you to use greater resistance by doubling up the band. This means there is more potential to avoid muscle loss in the glutes and hamstrings, which naturally weaken during menopause.

Reps: 12–15

Tempo: 1 second up, 1-second pause, 2 seconds down, 1-second pause

Progression: Use a thicker band

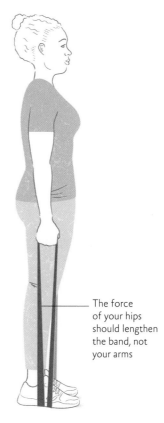

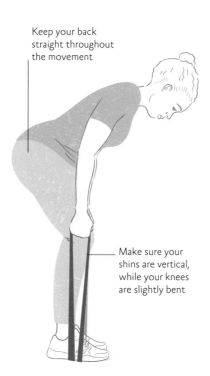

Keep your back straight throughout the movement

Make sure your shins are vertical, while your knees are slightly bent

The force of your hips should lengthen the band, not your arms

1 **Double-loop a band** and position tautly under the middle of both feet, your toes slightly turned out and your feet hip-width apart. Grip the ends of the band firmly. Push your bottom back as far as you can.

2 From a position leaning forward with a straight back—as if looking over a cliff—push your hips forward, squeeze your glutes, and stand upright. Hold, then slowly return to the start position.

BAND SPLIT SQUAT

As with the Supported Split Squat (see page 167), this exercise evens out strength, mobility, coordination, and balance discrepancies between your left and right legs. As muscle mass declines during menopause, it is beneficial to rebalance your body and improve your stability.

Reps: 8–10

Tempo: 2 seconds down, 1-second pause, 1 second up, 1-second pause

Progression: Use a thicker band

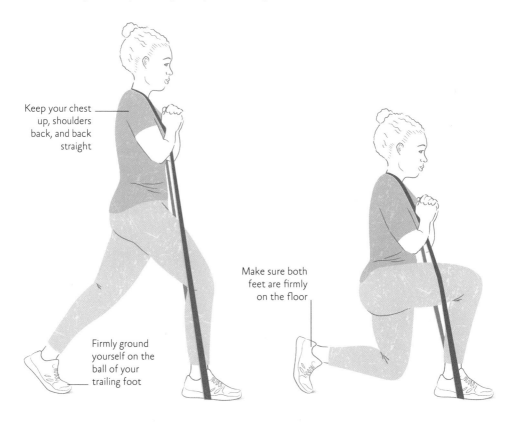

Keep your chest up, shoulders back, and back straight

Make sure both feet are firmly on the floor

Firmly ground yourself on the ball of your trailing foot

1 **Loop a band** around your front foot and the back of your neck with your feet at a distance that requires you to slightly bend your front knee. Position your hands in front of your chest with your elbows tucked in.

2 **Ensuring you are balanced**, descend in a straight line, bringing the knee of the trailing leg down to the floor. It can either touch the floor or stop just short. Hold, then drive through your front foot to stand.

HALF-KNEELING BAND ROW

This exercise allows you to train the upper to mid-back effectively by performing a simple pulling movement. As well as strengthening your back and challenging your biceps, it increases your grip strength and is great for improving overall posture, all of which can decline during menopause.

Reps: 10–12

Tempo: 1 second in, 1-second pause, 1 second out, 1-second pause

Progression: Use a thicker band

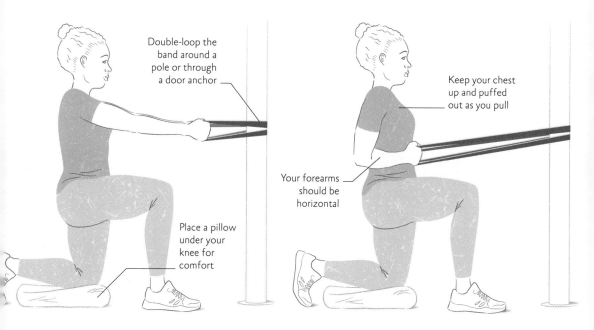

Double-loop the band around a pole or through a door anchor

Place a pillow under your knee for comfort

Keep your chest up and puffed out as you pull

Your forearms should be horizontal

1 **Anchor the band stably** to the height of your sternum in a half-kneeling position and evenly double-loop it. Grip the band and position yourself so there is slight tension in the band when your arms are straight.

2 **Leading with your elbows,** pull your hands into your stomach while squeezing your shoulder blades together— as if squeezing the juice out of a lemon. Hold, then return to the start position.

GYM WORKOUT

Using simple movements and easy-to-use equipment, this workout is a perfect introduction to training in a gym and lifting weights. It is particularly beneficial for menopause as it will develop your strength and help avoid the loss of muscle that commonly occurs. You can progress to this workout from the Bodyweight or Band Workouts (see pages 162–177), or start it immediately if you prefer.

WHAT YOU NEED

For the full workout you need access to a gym that has dumbbells, cable machines, and benches.

HOW TO FOLLOW THE WORKOUT

For best results, perform this workout—which takes around 45 minutes including the warm-up—at least twice a week, three times maximum, with at least one day's rest between sessions.

Some exercises have more than one version or a suggested progression. Start with the easier versions until you're confident.

- **Do 12–15 x Dumbbell Goblet Squats.** Rest for 30 seconds, then do 10–12 x Cable Crunches. Rest for 45–60 seconds. Repeat for 2–3 super-sets.
- **Do 12–15 x Cable Pull-throughs.** Rest for 30 seconds, and then do 10–12 x Seated Dumbbell Shoulder Presses. Rest for 45–60 seconds. Repeat for 2–3 super-sets.
- **Do 6–8 Dumbbell Split Squats** for each leg. Rest for 30 seconds and then do 10–12 x Seated Cable Rows. Rest for 45–60 seconds. Repeat for 2–3 super-sets.

SAFETY NOTE

To minimize your risk of injury, start with the warm-up (see page 161). If any of the exercises causes you pain, stop right away. Ensure that a fitness professional shows you how to use the equipment.

DUMBBELL GOBLET SQUAT

This adaptation of the Bodyweight Squat (see page 163) uses a dumbbell to challenge the strength of your legs throughout the movement. Because your muscle strength decreases during menopause, it is important to perform squats to help maintain your thigh muscles and improve mobility.

Reps: 12–15

Tempo: 2 seconds down, 1-second pause, 1 second up

Progression: Use the next-heaviest dumbbell

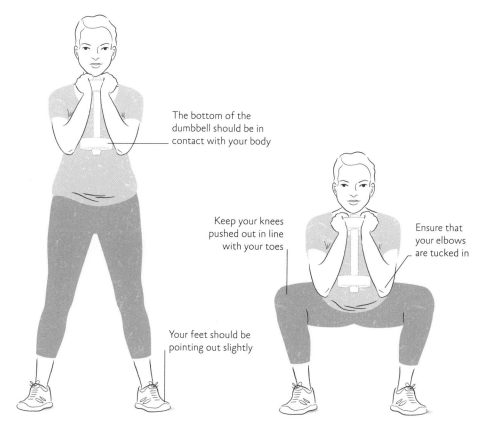

The bottom of the dumbbell should be in contact with your body

Keep your knees pushed out in line with your toes

Ensure that your elbows are tucked in

Your feet should be pointing out slightly

1 **Stand up straight** with your feet shoulder-width apart. Grasp the sides of the top end of the dumbbell, holding it so the top is in contact with the top of your chest. Press your forearms firmly into the dumbbell.

2 **Keeping your hands and arms** locked in position, sit back by bending your knees and hips at the same time. Descend as low as you can without your back rounding. Hold, then push through your mid-foot to stand.

KNEELING CABLE CRUNCH

This core exercise uses a cable station to strengthen the abdominal muscles, which can weaken during menopause and lead to lower-back issues. For maximum effect, compress your abdominals as much as possible when lifting the weight—like the bottom ends of an accordion being squeezed together.

Reps: 10–12

Tempo: 1 second down, 1-second pause, 1 second up

Progression: Use the next-heaviest weight

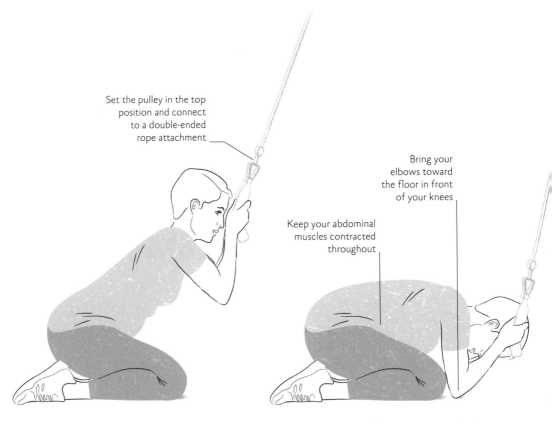

Set the pulley in the top position and connect to a double-ended rope attachment

Bring your elbows toward the floor in front of your knees

Keep your abdominal muscles contracted throughout

1 **Set the pulley and weight**. Grasp both ends of the rope and kneel down. Sit back onto your heels with enough room that your head will be around 12in (30cm) away from the weight stack at the end of the movement.

2 **Keeping your bottom** on your heels, contract your abdominal muscles and lean forward. Use the strength of your abs to lift the weight instead of pulling on the rope. Hold, then return to the start.

CABLE PULL-THROUGH

An excellent exercise for the glutes and hamstrings, this will strengthen your muscles, which may be weakened by menopausal changes. To ensure you are in the correct position, imagine you are peering over a cliff, with your bottom pushed back and your top half leaning forward.

Reps: 12–15

Tempo: 1 second up, 1-second pause, 2 seconds down

Progression: Dumbbell Romanian Deadlift (see page 182)

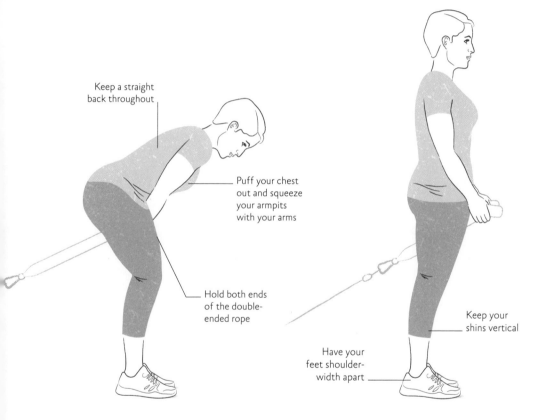

Keep a straight back throughout

Puff your chest out and squeeze your armpits with your arms

Hold both ends of the double-ended rope

Keep your shins vertical

Have your feet shoulder-width apart

1 Set the pulley and weight. Facing away from the weight stack, grasp the rope and step forward. Pushing your bottom back, lean forward, knees slightly bent. With straight arms, let your hands pass between your legs.

2 Pause—the weight should not touch the stack—then push your hips forward and straighten your legs to stand. The effort should come from your glutes, not your arms. The move should be a bow-and-arrow action.

DUMBBELL ROMANIAN DEADLIFT

This progression from the Cable Pull-through (see page 181) is a great strength exercise for sculpting and developing the back of your legs and your bottom, which may have become less firm during menopause. For correct positioning, imagine your body is following a bow-and-arrow action.

Reps: 10–12

Tempo: 2 seconds down, 1-second pause, 1 second up

Progression: Use the next-heaviest pair of dumbbells

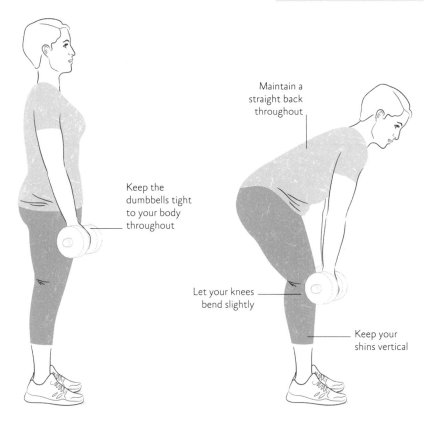

Keep the dumbbells tight to your body throughout

Maintain a straight back throughout

Let your knees bend slightly

Keep your shins vertical

1 **Keeping your arms** completely straight, grip a pair of dumbbells while keeping your shoulders back and chest proud. Tighten your abdominal muscles to keep your lower back flat throughout the movement.

2 **Push your bottom back** as far as you can, then lean forward with a straight back. The dumbbells should move in a vertical line toward the floor. Before your back starts to curve, drive your hips forward to stand.

SEATED DUMBBELL SHOULDER PRESS

This overhead pushing movement strengthens your shoulders and triceps. Keeping your arm, shoulder, and back muscles strong is important during menopause as the muscle mass declines, but regularly lifting weights above your head will prevent muscle loss and help with everyday activities.

Reps: 10–12

Tempo: 1 second up, 1-second pause, 2 seconds down, 1-second pause

Progression: Use the next-heaviest pair of dumbbells

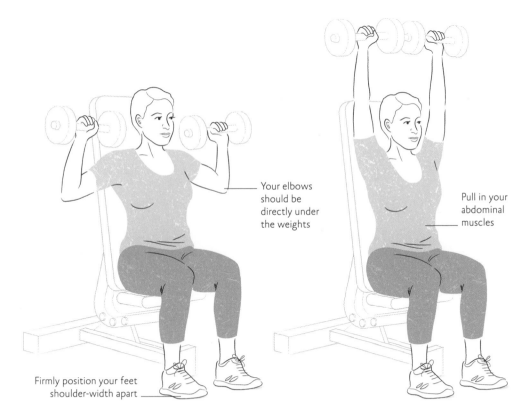

Your elbows should be directly under the weights

Pull in your abdominal muscles

Firmly position your feet shoulder-width apart

1 **Set up an adjustable bench**. Sit up straight with your back against the pad. Hold a dumbbell in each hand just above shoulder height, your palms facing forward. Your elbows should be under the weights.

2 **Drive your back** into the pad and keep your abdominal muscles tightened so that your back doesn't arch. Push the dumbbells toward the ceiling until your arms are straight and parallel, then return to the start.

DUMBBELL SPLIT SQUAT

This exercise is similar to the Band Split Squat (see page 176), but with dumbbells. It is a great exercise to do at menopause because it strengthens key leg muscles, aiding everyday movement. While the dumbbells provide a greater strength challenge, you may find that balancing is actually easier.

Reps: 6–8 per leg
Tempo: 2 seconds down, 1-second pause, 1 second up

Progression: Use the next-heaviest pair of dumbbells

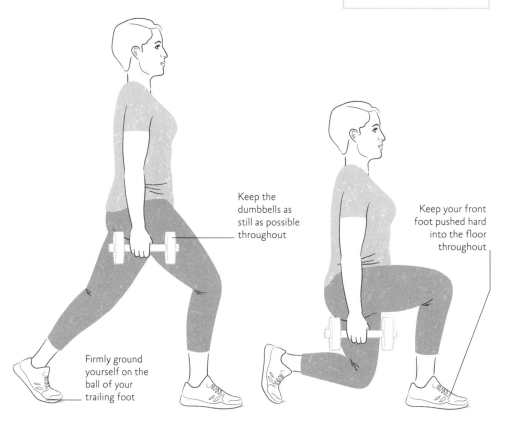

Keep the dumbbells as still as possible throughout

Keep your front foot pushed hard into the floor throughout

Firmly ground yourself on the ball of your trailing foot

1 **Grip a pair of dumbbells** by your side as if they were shopping bags. Keep your chest up, shoulders back, and back straight. Position your feet at a distance that requires you to slightly bend your front knee.

2 **Ensuring you are balanced**, slowly descend in a straight line, bringing the knee of the trailing leg down to the floor. It can either touch the floor or stop short. Hold, then drive through your front foot to stand.

SEATED CABLE ROW

Pulling movements such as the Seated Cable Row strengthen the mid- to upper back and maintain or even improve posture. A strong, upright back isn't just aesthetically desirable; it is essential to everyday activities and can help avoid impeded movement when the back muscles weaken at menopause.

Reps: 10–12

Tempo: 1 second pull, 1-second pause, 1 second release

Progression: Use the next-heaviest weight

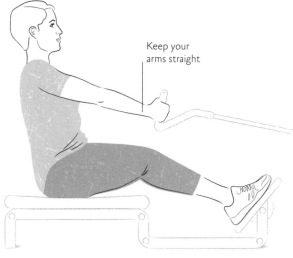

Keep your arms straight

1 Sit with your knees slightly bent, back straight, and chest up. Your feet should be pressed firmly into the foot plate about hip-width apart. Grasp the handles firmly and allow the weight to stretch your shoulder blades apart.

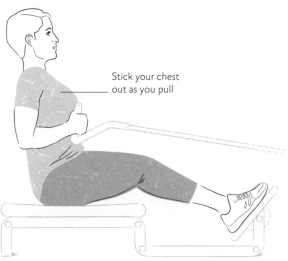

Stick your chest out as you pull

2 Smoothly pull the handles toward your stomach, leading with your elbows without leaning back. As you pull, keep your shoulders down and squeeze your shoulder blades together tightly. Then return to the start.

YOGA

Regular yoga—including restorative and supportive poses—will not only help create greater joint and tissue flexibility, but can also ameliorate the undesirable side effects of menopause. From fatigue to brain fog, anxiety, and insomnia, the sequence in this chapter (inspired by both yang and yin yoga) will encourage balance and peace of mind, providing both physical and mental stability.

WHAT YOU NEED
A calm, quiet space and a yoga mat. You may also wish to use yoga blocks and a bolster, but you can use rolled-up blankets or pillows.

FOLLOWING THE SEQUENCE
It's best to follow the order given here, but you can just choose a couple of poses that feel especially beneficial. During your practice, try to use the breath—lengthening on the inhales, and softening and relaxing on the exhales. Move between poses slowly and mindfully, especially going from seated to standing and vice versa. Find a level of effort that is "just right"; come to where you feel a stretch, then linger. Melt into that stretch. Time is more important than intensity.

If you wish, start with the modified version of the pose, and as your body relaxes, remove the prop and move deeper into the pose. Always use your breath to safely and effectively get progressively deeper and more relaxed within the postures—don't force anything.

The sequence will take around 30–45 minutes (or longer if you want). Practice as often as you wish, but ideally at least twice a week.

SAFETY NOTES
Be mindful and listen to your body. If you experience any pain or discomfort, try easing out of the pose a little. If the pain is persistent, stop. You may need to work with a teacher for correct alignment.

CAT/COW

Alternating between these two poses takes you through a range of motion that can benefit your back. By fluidly moving between Cat and Cow, you massage the joints and tissues surrounding the spine, which often get stiff during menopause, keeping them soft and supple.

Asana: *Bitilasana Marjaryasana*
Number of cycles: 5–10
Progression: Think about squeezing an invisible block between your thighs to engage the pelvic floor

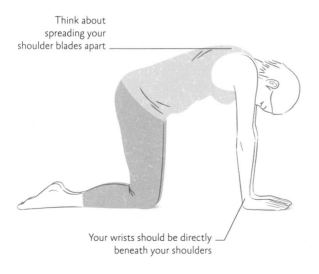

Your knees should be directly beneath your hips

Don't lift your chin too high

1 Start on all fours. As you inhale, broaden your collarbone and pull your chest through your shoulders. Slightly arch your back, keeping your lower abdominal muscles engaged. Press your head back, but do not strain your neck.

Think about spreading your shoulder blades apart

2 As you exhale, tuck in your tailbone and push the floor away to round your back. Relax your head and bring your chin in to your chest. Continue moving between Cat and Cow, working at your own pace and coordinating the movements with your breath.

Your wrists should be directly beneath your shoulders

LOW LUNGE

This posture stretches the hip flexors and the psoas muscles, deep-seated core muscles connecting the lumbar vertebrae to the femur. Menopause and its shifting symptoms can cause shallow breathing, but stretching the psoas muscles can free up your breath and release pent-up tension.

Asana: *Anjaneyasana*

Hold time: 5 slow breaths on each side

Progression: Do multiple rounds, trying to get deeper each time

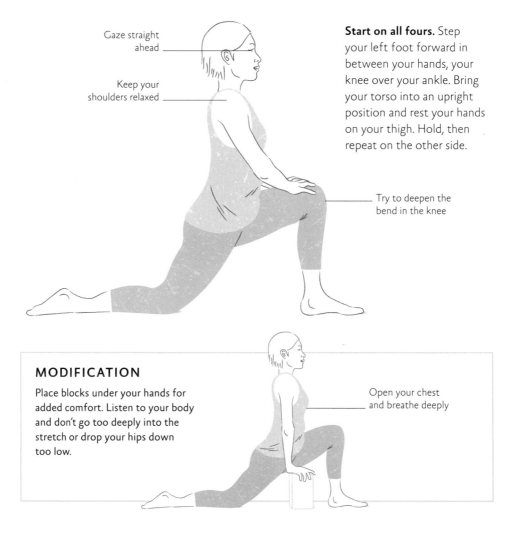

Gaze straight ahead

Keep your shoulders relaxed

Start on all fours. Step your left foot forward in between your hands, your knee over your ankle. Bring your torso into an upright position and rest your hands on your thigh. Hold, then repeat on the other side.

Try to deepen the bend in the knee

MODIFICATION

Place blocks under your hands for added comfort. Listen to your body and don't go too deeply into the stretch or drop your hips down too low.

Open your chest and breathe deeply

HALF SPLITS

This fantastic stretching pose increases awareness and stability through the pelvis. It may also help relieve joint aches and pains, which are common menopausal symptoms. You can pair it with the Low Lunge (opposite), inhaling forward into the lunge, then exhaling back into the stretch.

Asana: *Ardha hanumanasana*

Hold time: 5 slow breaths on each side

Progression: Do multiple rounds, trying to get deeper each time

Keep your chest and tailbone lifted to prevent your back from rounding

Make sure your hips are square

Start on all fours. Step your right foot forward in between your hands. Shift your weight back to straighten out your right leg and bring your hips directly over your back knee. Keep a small bend in the knee. Hold, then repeat on the other side.

Flex your front foot

MODIFICATION

Place blocks under your hands to help keep your torso erect and your spine lengthened. Bend the knee of the straightened leg more to increase comfort.

Try not to let your back round

189

RAGDOLL

Forward folds stretch the lower back, hamstrings, and calves, and this variation with the arms bound will bring relaxation to tired upper-back muscles. It will also help relieve tension in the neck, shoulders, and lower back—common complaint areas for a lot of women during menopause.

Asana: *Baddha Hasta Uttanasana*

Hold time: 1–3 minutes

Progression: Engage your quads and lift your tailbone to straighten out your legs

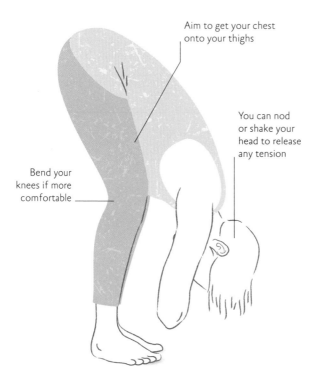

Aim to get your chest onto your thighs

You can nod or shake your head to release any tension

Bend your knees if more comfortable

MODIFICATION

If you find it hard to get your chest onto your thighs, increase the bend in your knees. You can also support your head and elbows with a block or a chair.

Keep your neck long—lengthen your head toward the floor

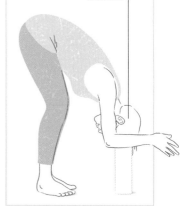

Stand with your feet hip-width apart. As you exhale, tuck your chin into your chest and slowly roll your spine down vertebra by vertebra into a forward fold. Clasp your opposite elbows with your hands, keeping your neck relaxed. Hold, then slowly roll up to standing.

WIDE-ANGLE FORWARD BEND

This pose stretches the insides and backs of the legs, as well as stimulating the bladder, liver, kidneys, and spleen. This pose will also help maintain the integrity and stability of the sacroiliac joints in the pelvis, which can become unstable during menopause as part of the natural aging process.

Asana: *Upavistha Konasana*

Hold time: 1–3 minutes

Progression: Walk your hands out in front of you and bring your chest all the way down to the floor

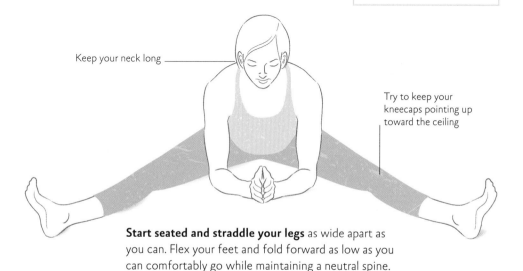

Keep your neck long

Try to keep your kneecaps pointing up toward the ceiling

Start seated and straddle your legs as wide apart as you can. Flex your feet and fold forward as low as you can comfortably go while maintaining a neutral spine. Hold, then use your hands to push the floor away and slowly roll up to seated. Bring your legs together, then shake them out to release any tension.

MODIFICATION

If your hips are tight or your lower back is excessively rounding, sit on a block or cushion to tilt your hips into a better position. You can also use a bolster or pillows to support your head, chest, and elbows.

Lift up through your chest

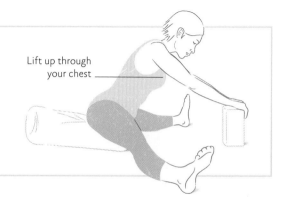

SHOULDER-SUPPORTED BRIDGE

This pose strengthens the lower back and stimulates the abdominal organs, lungs, and thyroid. It will help ease stress, fatigue, and insomnia and is therefore very therapeutic during menopause. To strengthen your pelvic floor muscles, you can also squeeze a yoga block between your thighs.

Asana: *Setu Bandha Sarvangasana*

Hold time: 30–60 seconds

Progression: Walk your shoulder blades together

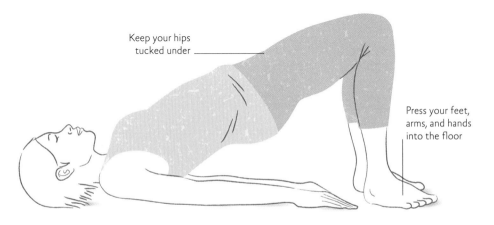

Keep your hips tucked under _____

Press your feet, arms, and hands into the floor

Lie on your back, knees bent, the soles of your feet hip-width apart. Bring your heels in close to your sit bones. Drive your hips up, until your thighs are parallel to the mat. Breathe in and out as you hold, then exhale and release, rolling your spine back down to the floor.

MODIFICATION

For added support, place a block under your sacrum/lower back. Try to squeeze your hips up away from the block, but rest back onto the block when necessary.

Adjust the block height to suit you _____

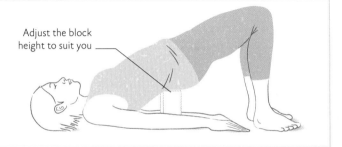

LOWER-BACK RESET

Though not officially a yoga pose, this stretch is fantastic to do after any type of back bend. It's also a good way to exercise your pelvic floor during menopause. Squeeze your pelvic muscles (as if trying to stop the flow of urine) while squeezing your bottom (as if trying to stop passing gas).

Hold time: 30–60 seconds

Progression: Once in position, rock gently from side to side

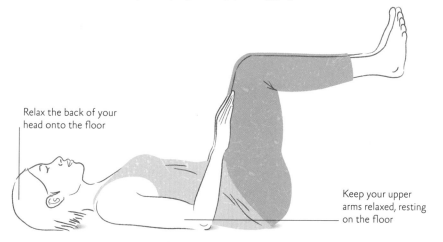

Relax the back of your head onto the floor

Keep your upper arms relaxed, resting on the floor

Start on your back in table-top position. Press your hands into your thighs at around 30 percent pressure, while at the same time pressing your thighs into your hands at 30 percent pressure. Engage your pelvic floor muscles. Feel your lower back lengthen and press into the floor.

MODIFICATION

If you can't fully engage your pelvic floor, squeeze a yoga block in between your thighs to help. If the position feels too intense, lightly rest your heels on a chair.

Keep your upper arms relaxed, next to your torso

RECLINED SPINAL TWIST

Supine twists are a fantastic tool during menopause because they improve spinal mobility and may aid sluggish digestion. Your posture will also benefit from this antidote to sitting down too much. This pose is best done toward the end of a practice when your body will be more supple.

Asana: *Supta Matsyendrasana*

Hold time: 2 minutes on each side

Lie on your back, legs outstretched. Bring your left knee in toward your chest. Place your right hand on your left knee and extend your left arm out. Exhale and gently twist your body. Gaze to the left and hold. Inhale to return to the start. Repeat on the other side.

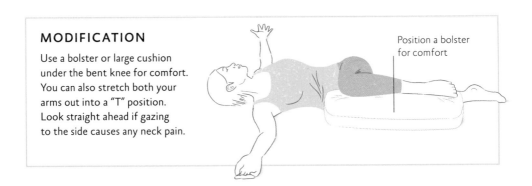

If comfortable, gaze toward the fingertips on your extended hand

With your hand, gently encourage your knee toward the floor

MODIFICATION

Use a bolster or large cushion under the bent knee for comfort. You can also stretch both your arms out into a "T" position. Look straight ahead if gazing to the side causes any neck pain.

Position a bolster for comfort

BUTTERFLY

This pose is calming and soothing, relaxing and quietening the mind, so it can be helpful when you're experiencing stress or menopausal hot flashes. It also stretches out your hip flexors, which get tight when you spend a lot of time sitting, helping relieve and prevent back pain and sciatica.

Asana: *Supta Baddha Konasana*

Hold time: Up to 10 minutes

Progression: Press your inner thighs to open up your hips

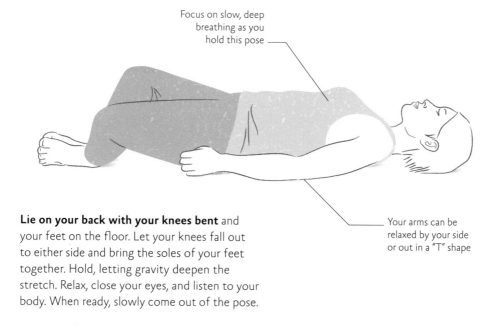

Focus on slow, deep breathing as you hold this pose

Your arms can be relaxed by your side or out in a "T" shape

Lie on your back with your knees bent and your feet on the floor. Let your knees fall out to either side and bring the soles of your feet together. Hold, letting gravity deepen the stretch. Relax, close your eyes, and listen to your body. When ready, slowly come out of the pose.

MODIFICATION

Use blocks or rolled-up blankets under your knees and/or pillows under your back and neck or head for support.

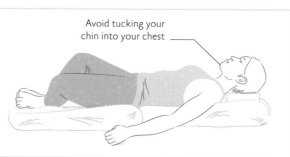

Avoid tucking your chin into your chest

LEGS UP THE WALL

This is a wonderfully relaxing and calming pose to do at the end of a practice or before going to bed. It can help bring relief to tired or cramped legs and feet, as well as calming the body and mind, which can often become stressed during menopause.

Asana: *Viparita Karani*

Hold time: 2–15 minutes

Progression: Widely straddle your legs if you want a deeper inner-thigh and hip stretch

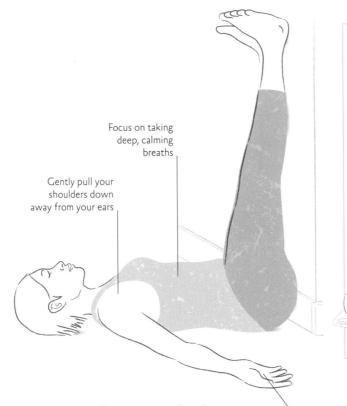

Focus on taking deep, calming breaths

Gently pull your shoulders down away from your ears

MODIFICATION

Place a small folded blanket under your head/neck for support. You can also move your bottom a little farther away from the wall, with your legs slightly bent, if it's more comfortable.

Close your eyes to promote a deeper state of relaxation

Lie next to a wall. Rotate around so that your legs go up the wall as your head comes away from it. Relax your shoulders and let your arms lie loosely. Hold, then when you're ready, fold your knees to your chest, roll to the side, and slowly come out of the pose.

Your palms can face up or down depending on which is most comfortable

ALTERNATE-NOSTRIL BREATHING

This calming but revitalizing breathing technique is ideal to do during menopause because it helps reduce feelings of anxiety and stress, as well as balancing your physical, mental, and emotional well-being. You can do it either at the end or start of a yoga sequence, depending on your preference.

Asana: *Nadi Shodhana*
Number of cycles: 5–10
Progression: Repeat for more than 10 cycles

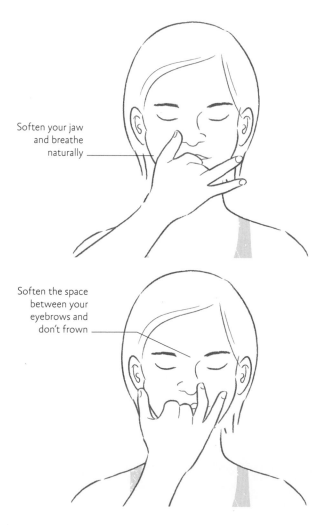

Soften your jaw and breathe naturally

Soften the space between your eyebrows and don't frown

1 **Sit comfortably**, ideally cross-legged. On your right hand, gently press your middle and index finger into your palm. Keep your thumb, ring, and little finger extended. Using your right thumb, close your right nostril and inhale as slowly as you can through your left nostril.

2 **Close your left** nostril with your ring finger. Pause, then release your thumb and exhale slowly through your right nostril. Inhale slowly back through your right nostril, then close it again with your thumb. Pause. Exhale through the left nostril. This is 1 cycle.

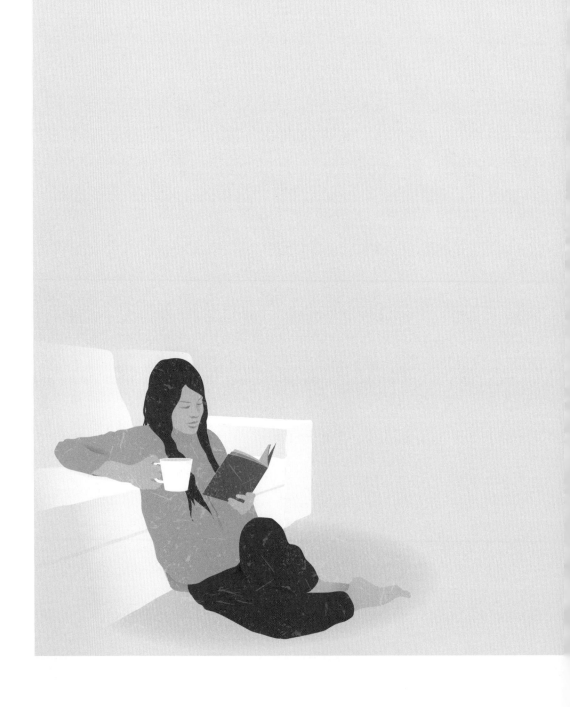

WHAT YOU NEED TO KNOW ABOUT HRT

INTRODUCTION

Many women have had concerns about using hormone replacement therapy (HRT). Nowadays, however, modern body-identical hormones have transformed the role of HRT during menopause. HRT will not only help many symptoms, but also confers long-lasting benefits to your skeleton and heart, in particular.

HRT involves the use of hormones such as estrogen, progesterone, and testosterone to replace the deficit in natural hormone production that occurs from perimenopause onward.

The main hormone responsible for the changes occurring at menopause is estrogen, specifically estradiol, which is the predominant form of the hormone produced by the ovaries in adult life. One of the primary aims of HRT is restoring estrogen to a level that is sufficient to manage menopausal symptoms.

In women who have a uterus, progesterone is also necessary to keep the endometrium (uterine lining) healthy and avoid any hyperplasia (thickening), which can be caused by taking estrogen on its own.

WHY TAKE HRT?

There are two key reasons for taking HRT. Firstly, HRT is an extremely effective way to reduce the severity of, or even prevent, many common but debilitating symptoms, from minimizing hot flashes, night sweats, and joint aches, to helping with insomnia,

brain fog, mood swings, and anxiety. See also pages 14–15.

Secondly, HRT can provide major health benefits, in particular for your bones and heart. Taking HRT long term can help maintain bone density and reduce the risk of osteoporosis, as well as reducing the risk of heart disease and stroke. See also page 202.

WHO TAKES HRT?

Some women will consider taking HRT when they are perimenopausal and have just started to suffer from symptoms, while others will wait until they are well into menopause or even post-menopausal. Some women will experience physical symptoms such as aching joints or digestive issues, while others will suffer from psychological symptoms such as low mood or anxiety. Unfortunately, some women will struggle with clusters of both physical and psychological issues, which can be debilitating. Although there are more than 30 recognized menopausal symptoms, it is rare for a woman to suffer from them all. See also pages 14–15.

“ ”

While you can take HRT for a short time to stop troublesome menopausal symptoms, the key point to be aware of is that this will not result in the long-term preventative benefits against osteoporosis and cardiovascular disease, which HRT can provide if taken for several years or even longer.

Some women will seek HRT even if they do not have any symptoms, but are aware of the potential benefits to overall health, while others may seek treatment as the result of debilitating symptoms.

HOW TO ACCESS HRT

If you are considering a consultation with your physician, it is best to go fully prepared. Use this chapter as a guide to the different HRT options available to help you discuss discuss which type of HRT will be best suited to you and why. There is also excellent information on the internet (see page 219).

While education and training surrounding menopause and HRT is becoming more common both for primary care physicians and gynecologists due to the endeavors of organizations such as the North American Menopause Society among others, this is still lagging behind the demand by women for expert advice and management and advice during menopause. Unfortunately, many doctors are not fully up-to-date with current HRT research, particularly as far as the risks

and benefits are concerned, which can lead to women being offered incorrect advice. If you feel this is the case, and you are not being listened to, you should ask for a second opinion or to be referred to a menopause specialist (see page 219).

Similarly, if you feel that the HRT you have been prescribed does not suit you, seek further advice and look at different types or strengths of HRT because the hormones frequently need to be tweaked or even changed more radically to ensure you have the best match for your individual situation.

Regardless of the HRT you are prescribed, it can take four to six months to ensure the regimen is optimized to provide control of your menopausal symptoms—with this approach it should be possible to produce around a 90–95 percent overall improvement in your well-being.

Prior to your first doctor's appointment, check that you are fully aware of your medical and family history, including details of the familial menopausal pattern, which can be a key predictor of your menopausal pattern.

THE BENEFITS OF HRT

Taking HRT can tackle problematic symptoms of menopause and can be life-changing for many women. It can also protect your bone and cardiac health and help increase both mental and physical activity, resulting in an improved quality of life and general well-being.

RELIEVES MENOPAUSAL SYMPTOMS

The most immediate and visible effect of HRT is that it can stop or reduce both physical and psychological menopausal symptoms. Initially—and often within a few weeks—HRT can relieve vasomotor symptoms such as hot flashes and night sweats, thus also benefitting sleep. Within a few months it can bring noticeable benefits to muscoskeletal symptoms such as joint aches and stiffness, as well as psychological symptoms such as anxiety, mood swings, and depression, which usually improve within three to four months of taking HRT.

PROTECTS BONES AND REDUCES THE RISK OF OSTEOPOROSIS

Taking HRT has been proven to prevent and stabilize the bone loss that occurs due to age and declining estrogen at menopause, even when taken at a low dosage. By maintaining good bone density you are at a reduced risk of developing osteopenia/osteoporosis and sustaining a fracture.

There is some ongoing protection against osteoporosis, even after HRT has been discontinued. Osteoporosis affects one in three women, and research has shown that bone loss accelerates in the years leading up to menopause, as well as the first two to five years immediately after periods cease.

HRT reduces the risk of both spine and hip fractures, and estrogen remains the treatment of choice for osteoporosis prevention in menopausal women, including those with premature ovarian insufficiency.

In addition to HRT, women should also ensure adequate dietary intake or supplementation of Vitamin D and calcium (see pages 141, 143, and 150–151) because these are vital for bone health.

SAFEGUARDS AGAINST CARDIOVASCULAR DISEASE

While there has been some debate about whether HRT is good for the heart or potentially harmful, HRT started ideally within 18 months of menopause can actually reduce your risk of developing cardiovascular disease, which includes conditions such as angina, heart attacks, and strokes.

Timing is key, and evidence points to a "cardiovascular window of opportunity," ideally within 10 years of menopause (when your periods stop), to achieve the optimum reduction in coronary heart disease and cardiovascular mortality.

CAN LOWER CHOLESTEROL LEVELS

Research has found that estrogen can maintain lower overall cholesterol levels and a healthy level of the beneficial HDL (high-density lipoprotein) cholesterol, which helps protect against arteriosclerosis and related problems.

HELP WITH ALZHEIMER'S DISEASE

At present there is conflicting research regarding Alzheimer's Disease, but there is some evidence from recent data that HRT may help reduce the risk of Alzheimer's Disease and other forms of dementia. The conflicting results are likely to reflect the importance of when HRT is started, and there may be a beneficial link to commencing HRT at an earlier age.

LONGEVITY AND IMPROVED QUALITY OF LIFE

Several studies show a reduction in all-cause mortality in women on HRT, when compared to both placebo and no treatment. This improved longevity is due to a variety of factors, including reduced morbidity from osteoporotic fractures and cardiovascular events, but it is also important to consider the overall improvement in quality of life that HRT can bring. This includes help with sleep disturbances and insomnia, musculoskeletal symptoms (such as joint pains and stiffness), mood instability, depression, anxiety, and cognitive function.

In terms of long-term health, HRT can also help with weight management and muscle retention, and may possibly help delay the onset of type 2 diabetes. Some of these outcomes are still being researched, but there is growing evidence for these benefits of HRT.

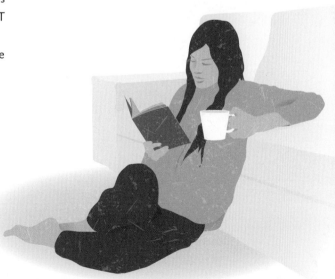

ASSESSING THE RISKS

Many women remain worried about the potential risks of HRT because the press has emphasized them in the past. However, current research is showing that taking the newer forms of HRT and starting treatment earlier, at the transition to menopause, can either reduce or eliminate these risks.

Most information leaflets accompanying HRT prescriptions include a long list of potential cautions to be considered before commencing treatment. Unfortunately, much of this information is outdated and has been superseded by more recent research. Many of the risks have been overblown or disproven and may have changed due to the availability of newer and improved versions of HRT. There are, in fact, very few women who should not take HRT as long as it is properly prescribed and monitored.

While HRT is generally very safe and highly beneficial for most women, it is important to understand the pros and cons of treatment so you can make a balanced decision about whether it is the right choice for you.

It is also important to consult with a health-care practitioner who has had appropriate menopause training and who can guide you to the best preparation for your individual situation.

There are three main risks that should be considered when starting HRT.

RISK OF BREAST CANCER

The risk of breast cancer is often the one that concerns women the most when starting HRT. This is understandable as there has been widespread coverage in the media about this risk, but this does not accurately reflect the entire literature on the subject. Plus, breast cancer is very common, with one in eight women likely to develop it in their lifetime, which makes it harder to determine what the underlying cause is in any one case.

Estrogen alone has not been shown to increase the risk of breast cancer. Even the large WHI study published between 2002 and 2020, which brought to the forefront the concern for cancer, has shown that there could be up to a 21 percent decrease in risk in women using estrogen alone.

The data about progestins and breast cancer is, however, more mixed, and it is thought that the real risk lies in the group of women on combined HRT, taking both estrogen and progestin. Many studies have pointed to an increased risk of breast cancer in patients on this regimen, although some studies have had major flaws, including the large WHI study.

Of key importance, the newer and more increasingly used body-identical micronized progesterone has impressive data showing its safety as far as breast cancer is concerned: a large-scale European study did not show any additional breast cancer risk for the first five years of treatment in women on combined HRT that included micronized progesterone.

RISK OF BLOOD CLOTS

Estrogen as a hormone is associated with an increased risk of forming blood clots in the veins of the body, most commonly the legs. This is true even of estrogen made by your own body.

Oral forms of HRT including estrogen are associated with a very small but definite increase in the risk of blood clots, but this is not the case with body-identical estrogen applied transdermally to the skin such as patches, gel, or spray, which are therefore a safer option.

CARDIOVASCULAR RISK

There is an increased risk of blood clot formation with age, which can also increase the cardiovascular risk of heart attacks and strokes. Other factors such as smoking, raised blood pressure, and high BMI also increase cardiovascular risk. There is some evidence that HRT may offset this risk, especially if commenced at the time of menopause and taken long term. Making healthy lifestyle changes in diet and exercise (see Chapters 4 and 5) can also help reduce this risk.

SIDE EFFECTS OF HRT

Most side effects have a limited severity and duration, and tend to resolve with time, particularly after six to eight weeks of starting HRT. So, if you do have initial side effects, it is worth persevering with HRT.

Some women can experience mastalgia (breast tenderness), abdominal bloating, indigestion, and headaches: some of these problems may be dose-related and can be minimized by starting HRT cautiously and building up the dose gradually.

In women with a uterus, unscheduled vaginal bleeding can happen in as many as 40 percent of women in the first four to six months of treatment and should not cause alarm in most cases. Where bleeding is either persistent, excessive, or unexplained, further investigations and specialized menopause advice should be sought.

A surprising number of women are also relatively intolerant to progestins and can develop symptoms that are similar to PMS. Fortunately, these tend to subside with time.

MYTHS AND FACTS

Many of the long-standing myths surrounding HRT come from older studies that have been either replaced completely or updated. It is important that you obtain information from a trained health-care practitioner who can address any concerns you may have and present an accurate view of modern HRT.

YOU SHOULD NOT TAKE HRT UNTIL YOUR SYMPTOMS ARE REALLY BAD

Whether or not to take HRT is an individual choice each woman must make for herself, taking time to balance the risks and benefits specific to her. Some women wish to explore all alternative options before starting HRT; others will decide to start HRT early on in menopause transition. Only you know which is the right choice for you, and if you have any doubts, seek advice from an experienced menopause specialist.

YOU CAN'T TAKE HRT WITH HERBAL REMEDIES OR SUPPLEMENTS

This is quite untrue and is one of the most commonly repeated misconceptions surrounding HRT. It is perfectly safe to combine HRT with any of the herbal remedies in Chapter 2 or the nutritional supplements in Chapter 4.

As HRT and herbal remedies work differently at the receptor level, they complement, rather than compete with, each other.

HRT WILL CAUSE WEIGHT GAIN

On the contrary, HRT has been shown to prevent weight gain. HRT can help you maintain muscle mass in place of fat, which is key to maintaining a healthy basal metabolic rate. It is particularly advantageous when combined with exercise such as strength training (see Chapter 5).

Some women may experience bloating and fluid retention, particularly in the early stages of taking HRT, but HRT itself will not cause long-term weight gain.

YOU DON'T NEED CONTRACEPTION IF YOU ARE ON HRT

As women start to transition into menopause it is tempting to assume there is very limited chance of conception, but this is incorrect. Until the age of 52, or when menopause is formally confirmed, it is best to use contraception if a pregnancy is not desired as HRT does not provide a high enough dose of hormones to give contraceptive protection. If unsure, seek advice from your health-care practitioner.

IF YOU COULDN'T TAKE THE PILL, YOU CAN'T TAKE HRT

HRT and oral contraceptives are very different types of treatments, and contain different estrogens and progestins, both in terms of formulation and strength. The doses used in HRT are significantly lower than those in oral contraceptives and are generally much better tolerated. Modern HRT prescribing has also seen the trend move away from prescribing synthetic hormones, such as those in the contraceptive pill, toward body-identical formulations.

YOU SHOULD ONLY TAKE HRT FOR A SHORT TIME

There is no scientific evidence to support the view that HRT should be taken in the smallest dose for the shortest length of time. This myth was based on concerns over the risk of thrombosis, breast cancer, and cardiovascular disease, but these concerns have been largely disproven with more modern forms of HRT and more recent robust studies.

The North American Menopause Society states that there is no set length of time or end date for HRT, and women should continue to use it for as long as it's beneficial.

HRT WILL DELAY MENOPAUSE

HRT does not change when women will go through menopause. While it may mask or stop menopausal symptoms, it is unable to delay menopause itself or alter the timing of it. Unfortunately, some women will continue to experience symptoms when they discontinue HRT. While symptoms that return at this time are usually of short duration, some women continue to have symptoms for many years after stopping Hormone Replacement Therapy.

YOU CAN'T TAKE HRT WHEN POST-MENOPAUSAL

Studies on various forms of HRT have shown that there is a safe window for starting HRT, which is up to 10 years from menopause. Some studies have shown that for maximum benefit in terms of protecting against cardiovascular disease, taking HRT up to five years into menopause is an ideal window.

HRT WILL CAUSE AWFUL SIDE EFFECTS

While some women have side effects such as breast tenderness and bloating, this is usually when they first start HRT, and problems tend to diminish after the first six weeks or so (see page 205). If you are experiencing persistent side effects, you are probably taking the wrong kind or strength of HRT for you and should discuss this with your health-care practitioner.

DIFFERENT TYPES OF HRT

There are three key HRT hormones: estrogen, progesterone, and testosterone, each of which can be administered in different formats, primarily transdermally (through the skin) or orally. The modern trend toward body-identical hormones is commonly associated with the transdermal route.

One of the original forms of estrogen used for HRT was conjugated equine estrogen, a blend of different estrogens produced from the urine of pregnant mares. Over the years concerns have been raised about the effectiveness of equine estrogens when given to menopausal women, as well as the ethical issues related to animal welfare. HRT such as this is therefore rarely used now and has been superseded by much more effective and safer forms of hormone therapy.

There is often confusion about the difference between bio-identical and body-identical hormones: compounded bio-identical forms of HRT are unregulated as opposed to FDA-regulated preparations available in a pharmacy, which are usually covered by health insurance. See also page 212.

WHAT KIND OF HRT WILL I NEED?

The type of HRT you require will depend primarily on whether or not you have had a hysterectomy, i.e. had your uterus removed (see box, opposite). The menopausal symptoms you are experiencing will also determine the most appropriate dose of hormones and whether additional hormones, such as testosterone, are required.

ESTROGEN

Estrogen can be prescribed via different routes and at a range of strengths. The most effective form of the hormone is estradiol, which is available as a skin patch, gel, spray, implant, or tablets for systemic treatment. Where local estrogen is required, this can be administered vaginally as a pessary, ring, or cream. See also page 210.

" "

It is important to be informed and find the right kind of HRT for you as an individual so that you can gain the maximum health benefits.

SINGLE VERSUS COMBINED HRT

SINGLE—ESTROGEN ONLY

This type of Hormone Replacement Therapy is used for women who have had a hysterectomy. Estrogen-only HRT can be prescribed on its own because progesterone is not needed to protect the uterine lining.

COMBINED—ESTROGEN AND PROGESTERONE

Estrogen and progesterone is prescribed for women who have a uterus as the estrogen helps to negate the menopausal symptoms while the progesterone protects the uterine lining from thickening due to the increased estrogen levels.

- **Body-identical estradiol** should ideally be given transdermally rather than orally, as this allows for more efficient absorption with reduced impact on bodily functions such as liver metabolism: this can be of key benefit because it removes the potential increased risk of high blood pressure or blood clots associated with oral estrogen.
- **Estrogen patches are** usually applied to the lower body, ideally the abdomen, and changed once or twice weekly.
- **Estrogen gel** is applied daily to the inner thigh, whereas the newest form of transdermal estrogen, the spray, is applied daily to the inner forearm. One of the main benefits of the transdermal forms of estrogen is the ease with which the dose can be modified to suit the individual. See also page 211.
- **Estrogen tablets** can be used for HRT. There are a range of doses available in estrogen-only and combined forms of these medications. There is only one dose of body-identical combined HRT for oral use. Given that the risk of blood clotting may be higher with these preparations, most women use transdermal forms. If you are better at taking an oral medication, there are options.
- **Local estrogen** can be administered locally into the vagina in the form of a pessary (a vaginal ring), cream, tablet, or gelcap. The main benefit of this route is that transfer from the vaginal tissues systemically into the bloodstream is negligible, and the impact of

the hormone is only exerted on the vagina, bladder, urethra, and other local tissues. Although local estrogen is a milder form of HRT, it can be extremely beneficial for symptoms such as vaginal dryness and discomfort and bladder problems such as recurrent cystitis, urgency, and frequency, but it will not treat the wider range of symptoms. Due to the lack of systemic absorption from local HRT, it is usually deemed safe, even for women who have experienced problems such as breast cancer.

PROGESTERONE

Most forms of progesterone used in HRT are taken orally, although some transdermal patches (which are combined—containing both estrogen and progestin) deliver the hormone through the skin.

Progesterone is required in women with a uterus to avoid undue thickening or hyperplasia of the endometrium when stimulated by estrogen. However, the local vaginal forms of estrogen contain much lower doses of estrogen than the systemic alternatives, which means that you do not need to use progesterone as well, even if you have a uterus.

Most progestins are ingested orally and historically have been synthetic in nature, which means they are more likely to be associated with symptomatic and metabolic side effects.

- **Micronized progesterone** is a newer form of progesterone and is a body-identical hormone. This form of progesterone is thought to be better tolerated from a symptomatic viewpoint than the synthetic versions, with fewer side effects, and also the benefit that it impacts on deep, non-REM sleep when taken at night, and thus helps improve the quality of sleep, which is a key menopausal concern.

Micronized progesterone also appears to be safer than the synthetic versions as far as breast cancer is concerned: a large-scale European study concluded that combined HRT, including micronized progesterone, did not increase breast cancer risk when treatment duration was five years or less, and although the data on treatment duration of greater than five years is scant, the incremental risks appear to be extremely small. This contrasts with concerns that progestins may increase breast cancer risk, although the studies are mixed on this topic, and it may have more to do with timing than the progestin itself.

- **The progestin IUD (sold as Mirena, Kyleena, and Skyla in US)** uses a synthetic progestin called levonorgestrel: while this is not a body-identical form of progesterone, the amount of progestin that travels from the coil through the uterine wall into the systemic bloodstream is thought to be almost negligible after the first six months of use. This means that the Mirena not only

THE MAIN FORMS OF HRT

ESTROGEN SKIN PATCH

This has been used successfully for decades and is easy to apply. The delivery route is not associated with an increased risk of blood clots or high blood pressure.

ESTROGEN GEL

This contains estradiol, which is also in the skin patch and spray. Although it is easy to change the dose, some women find the gel difficult to apply properly and compliance can become an issue.

ESTROGEN SPRAY

This is the newest form of transdermal estrogen and is probably one of the simplest applications to use. It is easy to vary the dose and dries in 20–30 seconds.

ORAL ESTROGEN TABLET

This is one of the original forms of HRT. Although well tolerated, oral estrogen is known to be associated with a higher risk of high blood pressure and blood clots.

LOCAL VAGINAL ESTROGEN

This is for women who mainly suffer from local symptoms such as vaginal dryness and discomfort, or pain during sex. It is a lower strength than other forms of HRT and is not absorbed systemically.

PROGESTERONE TABLET

Micronized progesterone is the newest form of progesterone. It is body-identical and is deemed to be safer and better tolerated than the synthetic alternatives.

PROGESTIN COIL

The Mirena coil is widely used. While it contains a synthetic progestin, it is well tolerated and is the only form of HRT that is also licensed for contraception.

ESTROGEN VAGINAL RING

An estrogen vaginal ring is used to give estrogen to the whole body—not to be confused with the lower-dose ring used just for vaginal symptoms. It behaves like a patch, and gives an even, constant dose of estrogen.

ESTROGEN IMPLANT

This compounded estrogen is not regulated by the FDA. It delivers a high and often uneven estrogen dose. It cannot be removed if there are side effects.

BODY-IDENTICAL OR BIO-IDENTICAL HRT

Body-identical HRT is also referred to as bio-identical HRT and is usually available by prescription from a pharmacy. The term body-identical is used to describe the fact that these hormones, once circulating in the bloodstream, are indistinguishable from the hormones naturally produced by the body prior to menopause.

Bio-identical HRT can be formulated from compounded hormones that are not regulatedby the FDA. Authorities such as the North American Menopause Society and the American Congress of Obstetricians and Gynecologists, among others, advocate against the use of this type of HRT due to safety concerns and other issues.

provides excellent bleeding control when used in HRT, but is also safer than oral synthetic progestins as well.

TESTOSTERONE

Testosterone is not an essential part of HRT for all women because the ovaries continue to produce low levels of the hormone even after menopause.

Occasionally testosterone is used for very specific indications; however, there are no female-dosed preparations available in the US. If you are using testosterone, this should only be done with a knowledgeable provider and with close monitoring to avoid side effects and harm from high dosing.

HRT IS YOUR CHOICE

Taking HRT is a choice each woman must make, taking time to balance the risks and benefits specific to her. Some women want to explore all of the alternative options before starting HRT. Some decide, based on the benefits (see pages 202–203) to start HRT early on in the menopausal transition. Only you know the right choice for you.

FINDING THE RIGHT HRT FOR YOU

It is important to work with your health-care practitioner to find the right type of HRT and correct dose for you. Your menopause advisor should take an individualized approach to ensure you obtain the desired results and maximum health benefits.

USING HRT HOLISTICALLY

HRT is one arm of a holistic approach you can use to improve menopausal symptoms and optimize health and well-being. When combined with good nutrition, exercise, mental wellness practices, herbal remedies, and aromatherapy, HRT can help throughout the menopause transition and beyond.

Many women who experience menopausal symptoms have already looked at their diet and their exercise regimen, undergone treatment for mental wellness issues, or tried herbal remedies. Often they are unable to achieve complete control over their menopausal symptoms even if they do their best to lead as healthy a lifestyle as possible.

If your sleeping pattern is disrupted or you are suffering from anxiety or debilitating hot flashes, you may find you are unable to solve these problems without considering HRT to boost your flagging estrogen levels.

If you are in a bad place because you have been suffering with menopausal symptoms for a long time—maybe you haven't slept properly for years, you have brain fog and are stressed about performing badly at work, or you don't have the energy to exercise, HRT may help turn things around. Without help it can be very hard to dig yourself out of a rut, and HRT can be the answer to help get your life back on track. As your health improves you may find that you finally have the energy to exercise more

or to explore mindful ways to de-stress. You may find that with improved sleep, cravings for unhealthy foods diminish, and you are able to focus on following a better, more nutritious diet. Sometimes, simply changing one key part of your life can produce a cascade that helps other areas.

HRT can be used alongside all the approaches covered in this book. In fact, maximum health benefits will be gained by using HRT while also evaluating and amending your diet, improving your exercise regimen, and incorporating weight-training on a regular basis, as well as using proven mental wellness practices.

In addition, herbal remedies and aromatherapy can be used either to help with persistent symptoms, or to maintain general health and well-being.

A holistic approach can boost the benefits of HRT and all the interrelated approaches work synergistically when combined together to help you maintain optimum health and happiness as you travel along your menopause journey.

BIBLIOGRAPHY

While every effort has been made to ensure that the materials in this book are accurate, the publisher apologizes for any errors or omissions and would be grateful to be notified about any corrections. All links checked September 2020.

CHAPTER 1: A NATURAL MENOPAUSE

British Menopause Society, www. thebms.org.uk

J. Murphy, "Ten post-menopause benefits to look forward to", *SAGA* [online], October 2015, accessed July 2020. www.saga.co.uk/magazine/health-wellbeing/wellbeing/10-post-menopause-positives

K. Abernethy, *Menopause: A Practical Guide to Understanding and Dealing with the Menopause,* Souvenir Press, 2018.

L. Earle, *The Good Menopause Guide,* Orion, 2018.

L. Newson, *Menopause,* Haynes, 2019.

M. Mathews, *The New Hot,* Vermilion, 2020.

Menopause Matters, www. menopausematters.co.uk

National Institute for Health and Care Excellence, "Menopause: diagnosis and management of menopause", *NICE* [online], accessed July 2020. www.nice.org.uk/guidance/ng23/documents/menopause-final-scope2

NHS, "Menopause", *NHS* [online], last reviewed August 2018, accessed July 2020. www.nhs.uk/conditions/menopause

R. Leonard, *Menopause: The Answers,* Orion, 2017.

CHAPTER 2: NATURAL REMEDIES

A. Ralph and G. Webley, "A prospective audit of pragmatic herbal treatment of women experiencing menopausal symptoms using measure yourself medical outcome profile (MYMOP2) questionnaires", *Journal of Herbal Medicine* 17–18, September–December 2019, 100286 DOI: 10.1016/j. hermed.2019.100286

A. Ralph and M. Tassell, *Native Healers:*

Foundations In Western Herbal Medicine, Aeon, 2020.

H. Brice-Ytsma and A. McDermott, *Herbal Medicine in Treating Gynaecological Conditions,* Aeon, 2019.

J. Green et al., "Treatment of menopausal symptoms by qualified herbal practitioners: A prospective, randomized controlled trial", *Fam Pract* 24, no. 5 (2007), pp468–474. DOI: 10.1093/fampra/cmm048

K. Bone and S. Mills, *Principles and Practice of Phytotherapy: Modern Herbal Medicine,* 2nd edition, Elsevier Churchill Livingstone, 2013.

S. Mills and K. Bone, *The Essential Guide to Herbal Safety,* Elsevier Churchill Livingstone, 2005.

036 Benefits of Herbal Remedies

G. B. Dudhatra et al., "A Comprehensive Review on Pharmacotherapeutics of Herbal Bioenhancers", *Scientific World Journal* 2012, (2012), 637953. DOI: 10.1100/2012/637953

037 An Herbal Approach to Menopause

B. L Fiebich et al., "Pharmacological studies in an herbal drug combination of St. John's Wort (Hypericum perforatum) and passion flower (Passiflora incarnata): in vitro and in vivo evidence of synergy between Hypericum and Passiflora in antidepressant pharmacological models", *Fitoterapia* 82, no.3 (2010), pp474–480. DOI: 10.1016/j. fitote.2010.12.006

P. J. Nathan, "Hypericum perforatum (St John's Wort): a non-selective reuptake inhibitor? A review of the recent advances in its pharmacology", *J Psychopharmacol* 15, no. 1 (2001), pp47–54.

038 Herbal Remedies versus Medicines

H. Wagner and G. Ulrich-Merzenich, "Synergy research: approaching a new generation of phytopharmaceuticals. *Phytomedicine* 16, no. 2–3 (2009), pp97–110. DOI: 10.1016/j. phymed.2008.12.018

J. Gertsch, "Botanical drugs, synergy, and network pharmacology: forth and back to intelligent mixtures", *Planta Med* 77, no. 11 (2011), pp1086–98.

DOI: 10.1055/s-0030-1270904

M. Wink, "Evolutionary advantage and molecular modes of action of multi-component mixtures used in phytomedicine", *Curr Drug Metab* 9, no. 10 (2008), 996–1009. DOI: 10.2174/138920008786927794

045 Lemon balm

A. Shakeri et al., "Melissa officinalis L. – A review of its traditional uses, phytochemistry and pharmacology", *J Ethnopharmacol* 2016, no. 118 (2016), pp204–228. DOI: 10.1016/j. jep.2016.05.010

H. Haybar et al., "The effects of Melissa officinalis supplementation on depression, anxiety, stress, and sleep disorder in patients with chronic stable angina", *Clin Nutr ESPEN.* no.26 (2018), pp47–52. DOI: 10.1016/j.clnesp.2018.04.015

M. Ranjbar et al., "Effects of Herbal combination (Melissa officinalis L. and Nepeta menthoides Boiss. & Buhse) on insomnia severity, anxiety and depression in insomniacs: Randomized placebo controlled trial", *Integr Med Res* 7, no. 4 (2018), pp328–332. DOI: 10.1016/j.imr.2018.08.001

047 Lavender

F. Algieri et al., "Anti-inflammatory activity of hydroalcoholic extracts of Lavandula dentata L. and Lavandula stoechas L", *J Ethnopharmacol* 22, no. 190 (2016), pp142–158. DOI: 10.1016/j.jep.2016.05.063

M. Nikfarjam et al., "Comparison of Effect of Lavandula officinalis and Venlafaxine in Treating Depression: A Double Blind Clinical Trial", *J Clin Diagn Res* 11, no. 7 (2017), KC01–KC04. DOI: 10.7860/JCDR/2017/20657.10233

M. Soheili and M. Salami, "Lavandula angustifolia biological characteristics: An in vitro study", *J Cell Physiol* 234, no. 9 (2019). DOI: 10.1002/jcp.28311

S. L. Chen and C. H. Chen, "Effects of Lavender Tea on Fatigue, Depression, and Maternal-Infant Attachment in Sleep-Disturbed Postnatal Women", *Worldviews Evid Based Nurs* 12 no. 6 (2015), pp370–379. DOI: 10.1111/wvn.12122

S. M. Hosseini et al., "The effect of aqueous extract of Lavandula officinalis to reduce cholesterol, triglyceride and other lipid metabolites on female BALB/c mice", *Clin Investig Arterioscler* 32, no. 3 (2020), pp111–116. DOI: 10.1016/j.arteri.2020.01.001

048 St. John's Wort
C. Stevinson and E. Ernst, "A pilot study of Hypericum perforatum for the treatment of premenstrual syndrome", *BJOG* 107, no. 7 (2000), pp870–876. DOI: 10.1111/j.1471-0528.2000.tb11085.x

M. D. van Die et al., "Effects of a combination of Hypericum perforatum and Vitex agnus-castus on PMS-like symptoms in late-perimenopausal women: findings from a subpopulation analysis", *J Altern Complement Med* 15, no. 9 (2009), pp1045–1048. DOI: 10.1089/acm.2008.0539

S. Canning et al., "The efficacy of Hypericum perforatum (St John's wort) for the treatment of pre-menstrual syndrome: a randomised, double-blind placebo-controlled trial", *CNS Drugs* 24, no. 3 (2010), pp207–25. DOI: 10.2165/11530120-000000000-00000

V. Briese et al., "Black cohosh with or without St. John's wort for symptom-specific climacteric treatment--results of a large-scale, controlled, observational study", *Maturitas* 57, no. 4 (2007), pp405–414. DOI: 10.1016/j.maturitas.2007.04.008

049 Chamomile
A. Ralph and G. Webley, "A prospective audit of pragmatic herbal treatment of women experiencing menopausal symptoms using measure yourself medical outcome profile (MYMOP2) questionnaires", *Journal of Herbal Medicine* 17–18, September–December 2019, 100286. DOI: 10.1016/j.hermed.2019.100286

A. Ralph and M. Tassell, *Native Healers: Foundations In Western Herbal Medicine*, Aeon, 2020.

D. L. McKay and J. B. Blumberg, "A review of the bioactivity and potential health benefits of chamomile tea (Matricaria recutita L.)", *Phytother Res* 20, no. 7 (2006), pp519–530. DOI: 10.1002/ptr.1900

K. Bone and S. Mills, *Principles and Practice of Phytotherapy: Modern Herbal Medicine*, 2nd edition,

Elsevier Churchill Livingstone, 2013.

S. Mills and K. Bone, *The Essential Guide to Herbal Safety*, Elsevier Churchill Livingstone, 2005.

S. Miraj and S. Alesaeidi, "A systematic review study of therapeutic effects of Matricaria recutita chamomile (chamomile)", *Electron Physician* 8, no. 9 (2016), pp3024–3031. DOI: 10.19082/3024

051 Skullcap
R. Awad et al., "Phytochemical and biological analysis of Skullcap (Scutellaria lateriflora L.): A medicinal plant with anxiolytic properties", *Phytomedicine* 10, no. 8 (2003), pp640–649. DOI: 10.1078/0944-7113-00374

R. Upton and R. H. DAyu, "Skullcap Scutellaria lateriflora L.: An American nervine", *Journal of Herbal Medicine* 2, no. 3 (2012), pp76–96. DOI: 10.1016/j.hermed.2012.06.004

053 Valerian
B. M. Dietz, "Valerian extract and valerenic acid are partial agonists of the 5-HT5a receptor in vitro", *Brain Res Mol Brain Res* 138, no. 2 (2005), pp191–197. DOI: 10.1016/j.molbrainres.2005.04.009

E. Jenabi et al., "The effect of Valerian on the severity and frequency of hot flashes: a triple-blind randomised clinical trial", *Women and Health Journal* 58, no. 3 (2018), pp297–304. DOI: 10.1080/03630242.2017.1296058

P. Mirabi and F. Mojab, "The effects of valerian root on hot flashes in menopausal women", *Iran J Pharm Res* 12, no. 1, pp217–222. DOI: 10.22037/IJPR.2013.1258

054 Oat Straw
K. A. Reynertson et al., "Anti-inflammatory activities of colloidal oatmeal (Avena sativa) contribute to the effectiveness of oats in treatment of itch associated with dry, irritated skin", *J Drugs Dermatol* 14, no. 1 (2015), pp43–48. https://pubmed.ncbi.nlm.nih.gov/25607907/

R. Singh et al., "Avena sativa (Oat), a potential neutraceutical and therapeutic agent: an overview", *Crit Rev Food Sci Nutr* 53, no. 2 (2013), pp126–144. DOI: 10.1080/10408398.2010.526725

055 Rosemary
J. R. de Oliveira et al., "Rosmarinus officinalis L. (rosemary) as therapeutic and prophylactic agent", *J Biomed Sci* 26,

no. 1 (2019), Article 5. DOI: 10.1186/s12929-019-0499-8

056 Licorice
C. C. Wang et al., "A randomized double-blind, multiple dose escalation study of a Chinese herbal medicine preparation for moderate to severe menopausal symptoms and quality of life in postmenopausal women", *Menopause* 20, no. 2 (2013), pp223–31. DOI: 10.1097/gme.0b013e318267f64e

L. Menati et al, "Evaluation of contextual and demographic factors on Liquorice effects on reducing hot flashes in postmenopausal women", *Health Care Women Int* 35, no. 1 (2014), pp87–99. DOI: 10.1080/07399332.2013.770001

P. Asgari et al., "A Clinical Study of the Effect of Glycyrrhiza glabra plant and exercise on the quality of life of menopausal women", *Chron Dis J* 3, no. 2 (2015), pp79–86. DOI: 10.22122/cdj.v3i2.155

059 Marigold
A. Ralph and G. Webley, "A prospective audit of pragmatic herbal treatment of women experiencing menopausal symptoms using measure yourself medical outcome profile (MYMOP2) questionnaires", *Journal of Herbal Medicine* 17–18, September–December 2019, 100286 DOI: 10.1016/j.hermed.2019.100286

A. Ralph and M. Tassell, *Native Healers: Foundations In Western Herbal Medicine*, Aeon, 2020.

British Herbal Medicine Association's Scientific Committee, *British Herbal Pharmacopoeia 1983*, British Herbal Medicine Association (2015), pp44–45.

M. Lievre et al., "Controlled study of three ointments for the local management of 2nd and 3rd degree burns", *Clin Trials Meta-Analysis* 28, (1992), pp9–12. https://eurekamag.com/research/008/387/008387217.php

S. Mills and K. Bone, *The Essential Guide to Herbal Safety*, Elsevier Churchill Livingstone, 2005.

060 Chastetree
H. Brice-Ytsma and A. McDermott, *Herbal Medicine in Treating Gynaecological Conditions*, Aeon Books, 2019.

R. Schellenberg et al., "Dose-dependent efficacy of the *Vitex agnus* castus extract Ze 440 in patients suffering from premenstrual syndrome", *Phytomedicine* 19, no. 14 (2012), pp1325–1331. DOI: 10.1016/j.phymed.2012.08.006

S. Mills and K. Bone, *The Essential Guide to Herbal Safety*, Elsevier Churchill Livingstone, 2005.

W. Wuttke et al., "Chaste tree (*Vitex agnus-castus*) – Pharmacology and clinical indications", *Phytomedicine* 10, no. 4 (2003), pp348–357. DOI: 10.1078/094471103322004866

061 Black Cohosh
R. Osmers et al., "Efficacy and safety of isopropanolic black cohosh extract for climacteric symptoms" *Obstet Gynecol* 105, no. 5 pt. 1 (2005), pp1074–1083. DOI: 10.1097/01.AOG.0000158865.98070.89

R. Uebelhack et al., "Black cohosh and St. John's wort for climacteric complaints: a randomized trial", *Obstet Gynecol* 107, no. 2 pt. 1 (2006), pp247–255. DOI: 10.1097/01.AOG.0000196504.49378.83

X. Ruan et al., "Benefit-risk profile of black cohosh (isopropanolic Cimicifuga racemosa extract) with and without St John's wort in breast cancer patients", *Climacteric* 22, no. 4 (2019), pp339–347. DOI: 10.1080/13697137.2018.1551346

062 Sage
M. Miroddi et al., "Systematic Review of Clinical Trials Assessing Pharmacological Properties of Salvia Species on Memory, Cognitive Impairment and Alzheimer's Disease", *CNS Neurosci Ther* 20, no. 6 (2014), pp485–95. DOI: 10.1111/cns.12270

M. Moss et al., "Aromas of salvia species enhance everyday prospective memory performance in healthy young adults", *Adv Chem Eng Sci* 4, (2014), pp339–346. DOI: 10.4236/aces.2014.43037

S. Akhondzadeh et al., "Salvia officinalis extract in the treatment of patients with mild to moderate Alzheimer's disease: a double blind, randomized and placebo-controlled trial", *J Clin Pharm Ther* 28, no. 1 (2003), pp53–59. DOI: 10.1046/j.1365-2710.2003.00463.x

S. K. Rad et al., "The effect of Salvia officinalis tablet on hot flashes, night sweating and estradiol hormone in post-menopausal women", *International Journal of Medical Research and Health*

Sciences 5, no. 8 (2016), pp257–263. https://www.ijmrhs.com/medical-research/the-effect-of-salvia-officinalis-tablet-on-hot-flashes-night-sweating-and-estradiol-hormone-in-postmenopausal-women.pdf

064 Red Clover
C. Atkinson et al., "Red clover derived isoflavones and mammographic breast density: a double blind, randomized, placebo-controlled trial", *Breast Cancer Res* 6, no. 3 (2004), R170–179. DOI: 10.1186/bcr773

G. E. Hale et al., "A double-blind randomized study on the effects of red clover isoflavones on the endometrium", *Menopause* 8, no. 5 (2001), pp338–346. DOI: 10.1097/00042192-200109000-00008

H. Fritz et al., "Soy, red clover and isoflavones and breast cancer: A systematic review", *PLoS One* 8, no. 11 (2013), e81968. DOI: 10.1371/journal.pone.0081968

T. J. Powles et al., "Red clover isoflavones are safe and well tolerated in women with a family history of breast cancer", *Menopause Int* 14, no. 1 (2008), pp6–12. DOI: 10.1258/mi.2007.007033

065 Maca Root
C. M. Dording et al., "A Double-Blind Placebo-Controlled Trial of Maca Root as Treatment for Antidepressant-Induced Sexual Dysfunction in Women", *Evidence-Based Complementary and Alternative Medicine* (2015), 949036. DOI: 10.1155/2015/949036

068 Aromatherapy Massage
F. Darsareh et al., "Effect of aromatherapy massage on menopausal symptoms: a randomized placebo-controlled clinical trial", *Menopause* 19, no. 9 (2012), pp995–999. DOI: 10.1097/gme.0b013e318248ea16

S. Taavoni et al., "The effect of aromatherapy massage on the psychological symptoms of postmenopausal Iranian women", *Complement Ther Med* 21, no. 3 (2013), pp158–163. DOI: 10.1016/j.ctim.2013.03.007

069 Clary Sage
P. Holmes, *Aromatica: A Clinical Guide to Essential Oil Therapeutics. Principles and Profiles*, Singing Dragon, 2016

W. Tarumi and K. Shinohara, "The

Effects of Essential Oil on Salivary Oxytocin Concentration in Postmenopausal Women", *J Altern Complement Med* 26, no. 3 (2020), pp226–230. DOI: 10.1089/acm.2019.0361

072 Sweet Fennel
F. Rahimikian et al., "Effect of Foeniculum vulgare Mill. (fennel) on menopausal symptoms in postmenopausal women: a randomized, triple-blind, placebo-controlled trial", *Menopause* 24, no. 9 (2017), pp1017–1021. DOI: 10.1097/GME.0000000000000881

M. Albert-Puleo, "Fennel and anise as estrogenic agents", *J Ethnopharmacol* 2, no. 4 (1980), pp337–344. DOI: 10.1016/s0378-8741(80)81015-4

M. Ghazanfarpour et al., "Effect of Foeniculum vulgare (fennel) on symptoms of depression and anxiety in postmenopausal women: a double-blind randomised controlled trial", *J Obstet Gynaecol* 38, no. 1 (2018), pp121–126. DOI: 10.1080/01443615.2017.1342229

074 Bergamot
X. Han et al., "Bergamot (Citrus bergamia) Essential Oil Inhalation Improves Positive Feelings in the Waiting Room of a Mental Health Treatment Center: A Pilot Study", *Phytother Res* 31, no. 5 (2017), pp812–816. DOI: 10.1002/ptr.5806.

075 Cypress
S. Battagia, *The Complete Guide to Aromatherapy*, 2nd edition, The International Centre of Aromatherapy, 2003.

077 Rose
K. Shinohara, "Effects of essential oil exposure on salivary estrogen concentration in perimenopausal women", *Neuro Endocrinol Lett* 37, no. 8 (2017), pp567–572. https://pubmed.ncbi.nlm.nih.gov/28326753/

CHAPTER 3: MENTAL WELLNESS

083 Understanding anxiety
ComRes, "BBC Radio Sheffield – Menopause Research", *ComRes* [online], December 2017, accessed July 2020. https://2sjjwunnql41ia7ki31qqub1-wpengine.netdna-ssl.com/wp-content/uploads/2018/01/J303687_BBC-Sheffield_Menopause-Survey_Tables.21.12.17.pdf

084 Personal Relationships
British Menopause Society, A woman's

relationship with the menopause is complicated...", *BMS* [online], October 2017, accessed July 2020. https://thebms.org.uk/wp-content/uploads/2016/04/BMS-Infographic-10-October2017-01C.pdf

084 Relationships at Work
Chartered Institute of Personnel and Development, "Majority of working women experiencing the menopause say it has a negative impact on them at work", *CIPD* [online], March 2019, accessed July 2020. https://www.cipd.co.uk/about/media/press/menopause-at-work

CBT
M. S. Hunter and M. Smith, *Living Well with the Menopause*, Robinson UK, 2021.

M. S. Hunter and M. Smith, *Managing hot flushes and night sweats: A cognitive behavioural self-help guide to the menopause*, 2nd Edition, Routledge, 2020.

M. S. Hunter and M. Smith in collaboration with the British Menopause Society, "Cognitive Behaviour Therapy (CBT) for Menopausal Symptoms", *Women's Health Concern*, 2017.

CHAPTER 4: NUTRITION
British Nutrition Foundation, www.nutrition.org.uk

L. Newson, *Menopause*, J H Haynes & Co Ltd, 2019.

M. Glenville, *Natural Solutions to Menopause*, Rodale, 2013.

P. Holford, *New Optimum Nutrition Bible*, Crossing Press, 2005.

122–131 Nutrition Introduction
A. Brończyk-Puzoń et al., "Guidelines for dietary management of menopausal women with simple obesity", *Prz Menopauzalny* 14, no. 1 (2015), pp48–52. DOI: 10.5114/pm.2015.48678

A. Valdes et al., "Role of the gut microbiota in nutrition and health", *BMJ* 2018;361:k2179. DOI: 10.1136/bmj.k2179

British Nutrition Foundation, Menopause, *BNF* [online], last reviewed November 2016, accessed July 2020. https://www.nutrition.org.uk/healthyliving/lifestages/menopause.html

British Nutrition Foundation, "Nutrition Requirements", *BNF* [online], revised August 2019, accessed July 2020. https://www.nutrition.org.uk/attachments/article/907/Nutrition%20

Requirements_Revised%20August%20 2019.pdf

British Nutrition Foundation, "Plant-based diets", *BNF* [online], 2019, accessed July 2020. https://www.nutrition.org.uk/healthyliving/helpingyoueatwell/plant-based-diets.html

British Nutrition Foundation, "Women: Top tips for women's health", *BNF* [online], last reviewed December 2016, accessed July 2020.
www.nutrition.org.uk/healthyliving/lifestages/women.html

J. L. Slavin and B. Lloyd, "Health benefits of fruits and vegetables", *Advances in Nutrition* 3, no. 4 (2012), pp506–516. DOI: 10.3945/an.112.002154

NHS, "Sugar: The Facts (Eat well)", *NHS* [online], last reviewed July 2020, accessed July 2020. https://www.nhs.uk/live-well/eat-well/how-does-sugar-in-our-diet-affect-our-health/

Nutrition Science Team, Public Health England, "Government Dietary Recommendations: Government recommendations for energy and nutrients for males and females aged 1–18 years and 19+ years", *PHE* [online], August 2016, accessed July 2020. https://asssets.publishing.service.gov.uk/goverment/uploads/system/uploads/attachments_data/file/618167/goverment_dietary_recommendations.pdf

Physicians Committee for Responsible Medicine, "A Natural Approach to Menopause", *PCRM* [online], accessed July 2020. https://www.pcrm.org/good-nutrition/nutrition-information/a-natural-approach-to-menopause

S. A. Lanham-New, "Fruit and Vegetables: The Unexpected Natural Answer to the Question of Osteoporosis Prevention?", *Am J Clin Nutr* 83, no. 6 (2006), pp1254–1255. DOI: 10.1093/ajcn/83.6.1254

S. Lecomte et al., "Phytochemicals Targeting Estrogen Receptors: Beneficial Rather Than Adverse Effects?", *Int J Mol Sci* 18, no. 7 (2017), pp1381. DOI: 10.3390/ijms18071381

132 Healthy Fats
H. Iso et al., "Intake of Fish and Omega 3 Fatty Acids and Risk of Stroke in Women", *JAMA* 285, no. 3 (2001),

pp304–312. DOI: 10.1001/jama.285.3.304

T. L. Psota et al., "Dietary Omega 3 Fatty Acid Intake and Cardiovascular Risk", *Am J Cardio* 98, no. 4A (2006), pp3i–18i. DOI: 10.1016/j.amjcard.2005.12.022

135 Protein
M. P. Lejeune et al., "Additional protein intake limits weight regain after weight loss in humans", *Br J Nutr* 93 , no. 2 (2005), pp281–289. DOI: 10.1079/bjn20041305

136 Carbohydrates
NHS, "The truth about carbs: Healthy weight", *NHS* [online], January 2020, accessed July 2020. https://www.nhs.uk/live-well/healthy-weight/why-we-need-to-eat-carbs/

137 Water
The United States Geological Survey, "The Water in You: Water and the Human Body", *USGS* [online], accessed July 2020. https://www.usgs.gov/special-topic/water-science-school/science/water-you-water-and-human-body?qt-science_center_objects=0#qt-science_center_objects

141 Vitamin D
Cancer Research UK, "Sun and Vitamin D", *CRUK* [online], last reviewed April 2019, accessed July 2020. https://www.cancerresearchuk.org/about-cancer/causes-of-cancer/sun-uv-and-cancer/sun-and-vitamin-d

National Institute for Health and Care Excellence, "Vitamin D deficiency in adults: treatment and prevention", *NICE* [online], September 2018, accessed July 2020. https://cks.nice.org.uk/vitamin-d-deficiency-in-adults-treatment-and-prevention

National Institute of Health USA, "Vitamin D Fact Sheet for Health Professionals", *NIH* [online], March 2020, accessed July 2020. https://ods.od.nih.gov/factsheets/VitaminD-HealthProfessional/

NHS, "The new guidelines on vitamin D – What you need to know", *NHS* [online], July 2016, accessed July 2020. https://www.nhs.uk/news/food-and-diet/the-new-guidelines-on-vitamin-d-what-you-need-to-know/

143 Calcium
S. A. Lanham-New, "Fruit and Vegetables: The Unexpected Natural Answer to the Question of Osteoporosis Prevention?", *Am J Clin*

Nutr 83, no. 6 (2006), pp1254–1255. DOI: 10.1093/ajcn/83.6.1254

144 Magnesium

J. J. DiNicolantonio et al., "Subclinical magnesium deficiency: A principal driver of cardiovascular disease and a public health crisis", *Open Heart* 5, no. 1 (2018), e000668. DOI: 10.1136/openhrt-2017-000668

149 Phytoestrogens

C. J. Haggans et al., "Effect of Flaxseed Consumption on Urinary Estrogen Metabolites in Post-Menopausal Women", *Nutr Canc* 33, no. 2 (1999), pp188–195. DOI: 10.1207/S15327914NC330211

C. Nagata et al., "Soy Product Intake and Hot Flashes in Japanese Women: Results from a Community-based Prospective Study", *Am J Epidem* 153, no. 8 (2001), pp790–793. DOI: 10.1093/aje/153.8.790

H. Adlercreutz et al., "Dietary phytoestrogens and the menopause in Japan", *Lancet* 16, no. 339;8803 (1992), pp1233. DOI: 10.1016/0140-6736(92)91174-7

N. Guha et al., "Soy isoflavones and the risk of cancer recurrence in a cohort of breast cancer survivors: the life after cancer epidemiology study", *Breast cancer Res Treat* 118, no. 2 (2009), pp395–405. DOI: 10.1007/s10549-009-0321-5

O. H. Franco et al., "Higher dietary intake of ligands is associated with better cognitive performance in postmenopausal women", *J Nutr* 135, no. 5 (2005), pp1190–1195. DOI: 10.1093/jn/135.5.1190

S. Rice and S. A. Whitehead, "Phytoestrogens and breast cancer – promoters or protectors?", Vol 13: Issue 4, Dec 2006. *Endocrinology* 13, no. 4 (2006), pp995–1015. DOI: 10.1677/erc.1.01159

150–151 Supplements

NHS, Vitamins and Minerals, *NHS* [online], last reviewed August 2020, accessed July 2020. https://www.nhs.uk/conditions/vitamins-and-minerals/

Nutrition Science Team, Public Health England, "Government Dietary Recommendations: Government recommendations for energy and nutrients for males and females aged 1–18 years and 19+ years", *PHE* [online],

August 2016, accessed July 2020. https://asssets.publishing.service.gov.uk/goverment/uploads/system/uploads/attachments_data/file/618167/goverment_dietary_recommendations.pdf

A. Ferrari, "Soy extract phytoestrogens with high dose isoflavones for menopausal symptoms", *J Obstet Gynaecol Res* 35, no. 6 (2009), pp1083–1090. DOI: 10.1111/j.1447-0756.2009.01058.x

British Nutrition Foundation, "Fact Sheet – Food Supplements", *BNF* [online], last reviewed August 2019, accessed July 2020. https://www.nutrition.org.uk/attachments/article/1259/BNF%20Food%20supplements%20factsheet.pdf

S. Sahni et al., "Protective Effect of Total Supplemental Vitamin C Intake on the Risk of Hip Fracture: A 17-year Follow-up from the Framingham Osteoporosis Study", *Osteoporosis Int* 20, no. 11 (2009), pp1853–1861. DOI: 10.1007/s00198-009-0897-y

CHAPTER 5: EXERCISE

154–185 Exercise Introduction and Workouts

B. Contreras and G. Cordoza, *Glute Lab: The Art and Science of Strength and Physique Training*, Victory Belt Publishing, 2019.

B. Schoenfeld, *Look Great at any Age*, Prentice Hall Press, 2003.

D. Segev et al., "Physical Activity – Does it Really Increase Bone Density in Postmenopausal Women?", *Curr Aging Sci* 11, no. 1 (2018), pp4–9. DOI: 10.2174/1874609810666170918170744

G. Slater, *Foundations of General Population Programme Design*, Lift the Bar Education.

J. Comas, "Top 12 Things Every Woman Should Know About Strength Training", *Girls Gone Strong* [online], accessed July 2020. https://www.girlsgonestrong.com/blog/articles/every-woman-should-know-about-strength-training/

M. L. Maltais et al., "Changes in Muscle Mass and Strength after Menopause", *J Musculoskelet Neuronal Interact* 9, no. 4 (2009), pp186–197. https://pubmed.ncbi.nlm.nih.gov/19949277/

N. Mishra et al., "Exercise Beyond Menopause: Do's and Don'ts", *J Midlife Health* 2, no. 2 (2011), pp51–56. DOI:

10.4103/0976-7800.92524

R. Lukas, "Is exercise an effective therapy for menopause and hot flashes?", *Menopause* 23, no. 7 (2016), pp701–703.

R. Zhao et al., "The Effects of Differing Resistance Training Modes on the Preservation of Bone Mineral Density in Postmenopausal Women: A Meta-Analysis", *Osteoporos Int* 26, no. 5 (2015), pp1605–1618. DOI: 10.1155/2018/4840531

Y. Lin and S. Lee, "Cardiovascular Benefits of Exercise in Postmenopausal Hypertension", *Int J Mol Sci* 19, no. 9 (2018), p2523. DOI: 10.3390/ijms19092523

186–197 Yoga

A. Swanson, *Science of Yoga: Understand the Anatomy and Physiology to Perfect your Practice*, DK, 2019.

H. D. Coulter, *Anatomy of Hatha Yoga: A Manual for Students, Teachers, and Practitioners*, Body and Breath, 2010.

H Cramer et al., "Effectiveness of Yoga for Menopausal Symptoms: A Systematic Review and Meta-Analysis of Randomized Controlled Trials", *Evid Based Complement Alternat Med* 2012, 2012:863905. DOI: 10.1155/2012/863905

N. Vaze and S. Joshi, "Yoga and menopausal transition", *J Midlife Health* 1, no. 2 (2010), pp56–58. http://www.jmidlifehealth.org/text.asp?2010/1/2/56/76212

S. Parkes, *The Manual of Yoga Anatomy: Step-by-step guidance and anatomical analysis of 30 asanas*, Quad Books, 2017.

CHAPTER 6: WHAT YOU NEED TO KNOW ABOUT HRT

National Institute for Health and Care Excellence, "Menopause: diagnosis and management of menopause", *NICE* [online], November 2015, updated December 2019, accessed July 2020. https://www.nice.org.uk/guidance/ng23/resources/menopause-diagnosis-and-management-pdf-1837330217413

H. Hamoda et al., "The British Menopause Society and Women's Health Concern 2020: Recommendations on Hormone Replacement Therapy in Menopausal Women", *Post-reproductive health*, 2020.

202 Bone Density

L. Zhu et al., "Effect of hormone therapy on the risk of bone fractures: a systematic review and meta-analysis of randomized controlled trials", *Menopause* 234, no. 4 (2016), pp461–470. DOI: 10.1097/GME.0000000000000519

202 Cardiovascular Disease

H. M. P. Boardman et al., "Hormone Therapy for Preventing Cardiovascular Disease in Post-Menopausal Women", *Cochrane Database Syst Rev* 3, (2015), CD002229. DOI: 10.1002/14651858.CD002229.pub4

J. E. Manson and S. S. Bassuk, "Invited commentary: hormone therapy and risk of coronary heart disease why renew the focus on the early years of menopause?", *Am J Epidemiol* 166, no. 5 (2007), pp511–517. DOI: 10.1093/aje/kwm213

R. L. Prentice et al., "Combined analysis of Women's Health Initiative observational and clinical trial data on postmenopausal hormone treatment and cardiovascular disease", *Am J Epidemiol* 163, no. 7 (2006), pp589–599. DOI: 10.1093/aje/kwj079

203 Cholesterol Levels

G. L. et al., "WISE Study Group. Hypertension, menopause, and coronary artery disease risk in the Women's Ischemia Syndrome Evaluation (WISE) Study", *J Am Coll Cardiol* 47, no. 3 (2006), S50-S58. DOI: 10.1016/j.jacc.2005.02.099

203 Alzheimer's Disease

C. Kawas et al., "A prospective study of estrogen replacement therapy and the risk of developing Alzheimer's disease: the Baltimore Longitudinal Study of Aging", *Neurology* 48, no. 6 (1997), pp1517–1521.

J. M. Matyi et al., "Lifetime estrogen exposure and cognition in late life: the Cache County Study", *Menopause* 26, no. 12 (2019), pp1366–1374. DOI: 10.1212/wnl.48.6.1517

L. H. Coker et al., "Postmenopausal hormone therapy and cognitive outcomes: the Women's Health Initiative Memory Study (WHIMS)", *J Steroid Biochem Mol Biol* 118, (2010), pp304–310. DOI: 10.1016/j.jsbmb.2009.11.007

203 Longevity

J. E. Manson et al., "Menopausal Hormone Therapy and Long-term All-Cause and Cause-Specific Mortality", *JAMA* 318, no. 10 (2017), pp927–938. DOI: 10.1001/jama.2017.11217

S. R. Salpeter et al., "Bayesian Meta-analysis of Hormone Therapy and Mortality in Younger Post-menopausal Women", *Am J Med* 122, no. 11 (2009), pp1016–1022. DOI: 10.1016/j.amjmed.2009.05.021

204 Breast Cancer

A. Fournier et al., "Breast cancer risk in relation to different types of hormone replacement therapy in the E3N-EPIC cohort", *Int J Cancer* 114, no. 3 (2005), pp448–454. DOI: 10.1002/ijc.20710

A. Fournier et al., "Unequal Risks for Breast Cancer Associated with Different Hormone Replacement Therapies: Results from the E3N Cohort Study", *Breast Cancer Res Treat* 107, no. 1 (2008), pp103–111. DOI: 10.1007/s10549-007-9523-x

Chlebowski et al., "Association of Menopausal Hormone Therapy with Breast Cancer Incidence and Mortality During Long-term Follow Up of the WHI Randomised Clinical Trials", *JAMA* 324, no. 4 (2020), pp369–380. DOI: 10.1001/jama.2020.9482

J. Rossouw et al., "Risks and benefits of estrogen plus progestin in healthy postmenopausal women: principal results From the Women's Health Initiative randomized controlled trial", *JAMA* 288, no. 3 (2002), pp321–333. DOI: 10.1001/jama.288.3.321

J. E. Manson, "The Women's Health Initiative trials of menopausal hormone therapy: lessons learned" *Menopause* 27, no. 8 (2020), pp918–928. DOI: 10.1097/GME.0000000000001553

205 Blood Clots

D. Rovinski et al., "Risk of venous thromboembolism events in postmenopausal women using oral versus non-oral hormone therapy: A systematic review and meta-analysis", *Thromb Res* 168, (2018), pp83–95. DOI: 10.1016/j.thromres.2018.06.014

ESHRE Capri Workshop Group et al., "Venous thromboembolism in women: a specific reproductive health risk", *Human Reproduction Update* 19, no. 5 (2013), pp471– 482. DOI: 10.1093/humupd/dmt028

RESOURCES

HERBAL REMEDIES

National Institute of Medical Herbalists, www.nimh.org.uk. The UK's leading professional body of herbal practitioners.

CBT

The Self Help CBT is available as a book: M S Hunter and M Smith, *Managing Hot Flushes and Night Sweats: A cognitive behavioural Self-help Guide to the menopause.* 2nd Edition, Routledge, 2020. www.routledge.com

Fact Sheets on CBT for women and for health professionals are available on the Women's Health Concern website: www.womens-health-concern.org

Try www.findcbt.org/FAT/ and www.psychologytoday.com/us/therapists/cognitive-behavioral-cbt.There is a free app called "CBTi" for insomnia, developed for veterans with PTSD through the VA.

For a private CBT therapist, the Association for Behavioral and Cognitive Therapies has a helpful website (www.abct.org) that includes a register of accredited CBT therapists in the US and Canada.

NUTRITION

For recommended daily intake of key vitamins and minerals see: www.nutrition.gov/topics/whats-food/vitamins-and-minerals

HRT

The North American Menopause Society has a helpful website, www.abct.org and a includes a database for finding a specialist near you: portal.menopause.org/NAMS/NAMS/Directory/Menopause-Practitioner.aspx

INDEX

ABOUT THE AUTHORS

Anne Henderson MA MB BChir MRCOG (Consulting Editor and HRT) is a consultant gynecologist and BMS-accredited menopause expert with over thirty years' experience in menopause, running clinics in the United Kingdom. She is an advocate for holistic menopause care and is also an advocate for complementary therapies and nutrition for all her menopausal patients. Anne undertook her medical studies at Cambridge University and currently runs a busy women's health clinic, The Amara Clinic, in Kent, United Kingdom. www.gynae-expert.co.uk

Rebecca Dunsmoor-Su MD, MSCE NCMP (US Consulting Editor and HRT) is a NAMS-certified menopause practitioner and the Medical Director for Menopause at Swedish Medical Center/Providence Health System in Seattle, Washington. She is also the Chief Medical Officer for Gennev.com, the leading online clinical resource for women in midlife and menopause.

Anita Ralph MSc (herb med) MNIMH MCPP (Herbal Remedies) is a consulting medical herbalist and cofounded the first Integrated Gynecology Clinic in the UK. She is a lecturer and author of a foundation course and textbook for herbal medicine. www.medicinetreeherbs.co.uk

Louise Robinson (Essential Oils) is a therapist with qualifications in aromatherapy, massage, and reflexology. She runs a thriving therapy practice and works with the NHS. She is passionate about helping her clients through holistic therapeutic treatments. www.louiserobinson.co.uk

Diane Danzebrink (Mental Wellness) is a Menopause Counselor and expert working in private practice. She is the founder of the nonprofit organization Menopause Support menopausesupport.co.uk and the #MakeMenopauseMatter campaign. www.dianedanzebrink.com

Dr. Myra Hunter (CBT) is Emeritus Professor of clinical health psychology at the Institute of Psychiatry, Psychology, and Neuroscience, King's College London. She has developed effective cognitive behavioral interventions for menopausal symptoms.

Sabrina Zeif (Nutrition) is The Midlife Food Guru. Nutritional therapist, chef, host, and founder of The Menopause Chef, she approaches food and nutrition as she does life: celebrate and savor! www.midlifefoodguru.com

Paul Harter (Exercise) is a retired law firm partner. At age 60, he became a personal trainer and certified nutritionist. He founded Goal Master, a leading London-based provider of fitness, nutrition, and lifestyle coaching for busy people. www.goalmasterfitness.com

Don Graham (Exercise) is Head of Coaching at Goal Master and an active participant in the evidence-based fitness community. He specializes in helping professionals create sustainable health-focused lifestyles.

Lauren Halsey (Exercise) is a Senior Coach at Goal Master. She is a personal trainer, yoga instructor, and mobility specialist. She is an expert at coaching women through their menopause journey.

ACKNOWLEDGMENTS

Consulting Editor: Thank you to all the expert contributors and the team at DK who were enormously supportive during the writing of this book, particularly Claire Wedderburn-Maxwell and Dawn Henderson, as well as the highly talented design team who have produced the wonderful layout.
DK: Thank you to Jane Ellis for proofreading; Hilary Bird for creating the index; and Tom Moore for his technical support.